Animal Toxicity Studies: Their Relevance for Man

CMR Workshop Series

Monitoring for Adverse Drug Reactions
Editors: S.R. Walker and A. Goldberg

Long-Term Animal Studies
Their Predictive Value for Man
Editors: S.R. Walker and A.D. Dayan

Medicines and Risk/Benefit Decisions
Editors: S.R. Walker and A.W. Asscher

Quality of Life: Assessment and Application
Editors: S.R. Walker and R.M. Rosser

International Medicines Regulations
A Forward Look to 1992
Editors: S.R. Walker and J.P Griffin

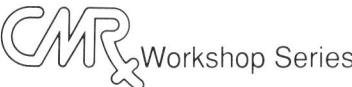Workshop Series

Animal Toxicity Studies: Their Relevance for Man

EDITED BY

C.E. Lumley

S.R. Walker

*Proceedings of a Workshop
held at
The Ciba Foundation
London, UK
26th September 1989*

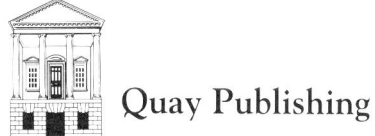Quay Publishing

Quay Pubishing
11 Victoria Wharf
St Georges Quay
Lancaster LA1 1GA

British Library Cataloguing in Publication Data
Lumley, C.E. (Cindy E.)
  Animal toxicity studies: their relevance for man.
  1. Medicine. Research. Use of laboratory animals
  I. Title. II. Walker, S.R. (Stuart Russell)   1944–
  619

ISBN 1-85642-000-0

© 1990 by Quay Publishing

All rights reserved. No part of this publication may be reproduced, stored in a retrieval system, or transmitted in any form or by any means, electronic, mechanical, photocopying, recording or otherwise, without prior permission from the publishers.

Laserprinter typeset by Martin Lister Publishing Services, Bolton-le-Sands, Lancs.
Printed in Great Britain by Butler & Tanner Limited, Frome and London

Contents

Preface		vii
Notes on contributors		ix

I. Setting the Scene

1. Expectations from animal studies
   D. Morton — 3

2. The importance of retrospective comparisons
   R. Brimblecombe — 15

II. Methodology: A Critical Appraisal
A. The Global Approach

3. Antineoplastics, a unique group
   P. Schein — 23

4. What can be learnt by examining the data in the files of regulatory authorities? – a toxicologist's viewpoint
   R. Bass — 33

5. What can be learnt by examining the data in the files of regulatory authorities? – a clinician's viewpoint
   P. Fletcher — 41

B. Clinical Toxicity - Could it have been Predicted?

6. Clinical toxicity - could it have been predicted? Pre-marketing experience
   C.E. Lumley — 49

7. Clinical toxicity – could it have been predicted? Post-marketing experience
   R. Heywood — 57

C. What can be Learnt from Case Studies?

8. The company approach
   K. Suter — 71

9. A collaborative approach
   A. McLean — 79

III. Recommendations for Future Work: Summary of Discussion

10. Recommendations for future work: summary of discussion
    C.E. Lumley and S.R. Walker — 85

Index — 91

Preface

There are powerful scientific, ethical and regulatory reasons for exploring the effects of potential therapeutic candidates in animals before they are administered to man. The low proportion of significant toxic reactions in humans with new medicines, compared to the number tested and introduced, supports the contention that toxicity studies in laboratory animals are, in the main, predictive for man. There are also many concurrences between the findings in animal toxicity tests and adverse reactions in humans, particularly for dose- and time-related toxic effects. On the other hand, there have been well-publicised failures of experimental toxicology and false alarms resulting from apparently irrelevant toxicological observations in animals.

The overall success of the current preclinical safety evaluation process is difficult to assess. Although useful information can be obtained by retrospective analysis of data obtained for compounds that have been used extensively in the clinic, to date this has received little systematic study. The sixth CMR Workshop provided the opportunity for an international group of experts from the pharmaceutical industry, academia and the regulatory authorities to critically review and discuss past methodologies which have been employed to assess the efficacy of the animal toxicity testing procedure in predicting qualitative toxicity in man. It is hoped that the recommendations made will give rise to a new programme of research, aimed at studying the correlation between animal and clinical data, in order to improve future predictions and risk assessment, and to identify areas where basic research is needed.

The publication of the proceedings of this Workshop would not have been possible without a considerable amount of work and support by the Centre's staff. In particular, the Editors wish to thank Miss Julie Winch for so capably handling the administration arrangements for this meeting, and for her secretarial support. Finally, our thanks are due to all the participants who made the sixth CMR Workshop such a success.

Dr Cyndy E. Lumley
Professor Stuart R. Walker
June 1990

Notes on Contributors

Professor R Bass MD is Head of Toxicology, Director and Professor at the Institute for Drugs of the Federal Health Office, Berlin. Since 1984 he has been Adjunct Professor of Pharmacology and Toxicology at the Free University, Berlin. Todays research interests are in reproduction and short-term tests in toxicology. He has published over 90 papers, articles and books in these areas and on formaldehyde, animal experiments and protection and regulatory toxicology.

Dr R Brimblecombe DSc, FRCPATH is Vice-President, Collaborative Research and Development (Worldwide) for Smith Kline & French Laboratories. He has held a series of senior positions in SK&F R&D since 1973. A pharmacologist by training he has developed an increasing interest in toxicology, especially in the predictiveness of animal studies for effects in man.

Dr P Fletcher MB, PhD, Medical Director, IMS International.

Dr R Heywood PhD, Dr Med. Vet., BVMS, FRCPath, MRCVS, FIBiol. has been involved with comparative laboratory animal medicine and pathology for 30 years and with toxicological studies for 25 years. He was Scientific Director of the Huntingdon Research Centre and is currently an Independent Consultant in Toxicology. He is the author of over 150 research papers in toxicology.

Dr C E Lumley BSc, PhD is Project Manager at the Centre for Medicines Re search. Her current research interests include safety testing of new medicines, drug regulations, the predictive value of animal studies for man and pharmaceutical Research and Development expenditure. Dr Lumley is a regular contributor to Scientific Journals and Meetings.

Professor A E M McLean BM, BCH(Oxon), PhD(Lond), FRCPath, is First Professor of Toxicology at the University of London. He previously worked for the Medical Research Council in their Toxi-

Notes on Contributors

cology Research Unit and in their West Indies unit on problems of malnutrition and toxicity. Professor McLean is interested in the relationship between nutrition and biochemical pathways leading to toxicity, and in the use of epidemiological methods to verify laboratory findings and has research projects on mechanisms of recovery from cell injury and nutritional factors in intestinal cancer.

Dr D M Morton BPharm, PhD, CChem, MRSC, MRPS, is Vice-President of Lilly Research Laboratories and Professor of Pharmacology and Toxicology at the Indiana University School of Medicine. Prior to his current appointment, he held several research positions at Lilly in both England and the United States. His areas of research interest include pharmacology, drug metabolism and toxicology and he is the author of thirty research papers.

Dr P S Schein MD, FRCP is currently President and Chief Executive Officer at U.S. Bioscience, Inc. and Adjunct Professor of Medicine and Pharmacology at the University of Pennsylvania School of Medicine. Formerly, he was Scientific Director of the Lombardi Cancer Research Center, Chairman of the FDA's Advisory Committee for Oncologic Drugs and President of the American Society of Clinical Oncology. He has authored over 300 research papers and books in the fields of pharmacology and oncology.

Dr K E Suter is head of the Sandoz Reproduction Toxicology Section and has a broad interest in the safety aspects of drugs and chemicals. After postdoctoral training in the USA in the field of chemical mutagenesis he entered the preclinical research department of Sandoz Ltd. in 1975.

Professor S R Walker BSc, PhD, CChem, FRSC, CBiol, FIBiol is Director of the Centre for Medicines Research and Honorary Professor of the Welsh School of Pharmacy, Cardiff. His current research involves an assessment of the innovation and development of new medicines, investigating the predictive value of preclinical animal toxicology, improving the methodology for assessing quality of life in the determination of the benefits of medicines and the evaluation of post-marketing surveillance schemes. He is the author of over 100 research papers and six books.

I.
Setting the Scene

1
Expectations from animal studies

DOUG MORTON

Summary

1. The protocols of toxicity tests and accompanying metabolism and pharmacokinetic studies have evolved successfully due to careful comparisons with clinical experience in man.
2. Animal studies should adequately characterise the toxicity of a new medicine in several species, so that the clinician can be alerted to possible similar effects in man.
3. Evidence is presented, from the literature and from an analysis of compounds tested by the Lilly Research Laboratories, to support the conclusion that the absence of a carcinogenic response in long-term rodent studies can provide a significant measure of confidence to proceed with the development of a new drug for chronic therapy.
4. The low proportion of significant toxic reactions in humans with new drugs, compared to the number tested and introduced, supports the contention that toxicity studies in laboratory animals are, in the main, predictive for man.

Introduction

The development of potent and effective drugs continues to be associated with a concern regarding their safety. The administration of biologically active compounds to man must always be accompanied by some element of risk that cannot be avoided by even the most careful and exhaustive scientific study of the drug in animals before it is introduced. The decision to introduce a new drug depends on the balance between clinical benefit and risk, with the risk assessment usually involving determination of toxic and "no adverse effect doses" in laboratory animals. All compounds can be toxic in overdosage and, even in their therapeutic range, many useful drugs have unavoidable toxic side-effects.

The wide-range of valuable therapeutic agents which have gained clinical acceptance and government regulatory approval attests to the predictability of pharmacological and toxicological studies in animals. The protocols of toxicity tests and accompanying metabolism and pharmacokinetic studies have evolved successfully due to careful comparisons with man clinical experience. A detailed listing of the toxic reactions produced by chemicals that have occurred in both laboratory animals and man was presented by Zbinden[1] in the Centre for Medicines Research Annual Lecture in 1987 (Table 1). The amount of comparative data has, of course, been limited since compounds that produce significant toxicity in laboratory animals do not normally progress to clinical testing in humans.

Table 1. A selection of toxic reactions occuring in animals and man

Acetaminophen	Hepatic necrosis
Acrylamide	Peripheral neuropathy
Aniline	Methaemoglobinaemia
Asbestos	Mesothelioma
Atropine	Constipation
Benzene	Leukaemia
Bleomycin	Pulmonary fibrosis
Carbon disulphide	Nervous system toxicity
Carbon tetrachloride	Hepatic necrosis
Cis-platinum	Nephropathy

Table 1 (continued)

Cobalt sulphate	Cardiomyopathy
Cyclophosphamide	Haemorrhagic cystitis
Cyclosporin A	Nephropathy
D&C Yellow	Eczema
Diethylene glycol	Nephropathy
Diethylaminoethoxyhexoestrol	Phospholipidosis of liver
Doxorubicin	Cardiomyopathy
Emetine	ECG abnormalities
Ethylene glycol	Obstructive nephropathy
Furosemide	Hypokalaemia
Gentamycin	Nephropathy
Hexacarbons	Peripheral neuropathy
Hexachlorophene	Spongiforme encephalopathy
Isoniazid	Peripheral neuropathy
Isoproterenol	Stenocardia
Isothiocyanates	Goitre
Isotretinoin, prenatal	Multiple malformations
Kanamycin	Cochlear toxicity
Methanol	Blindness (monkey)
Methoxyflurane	Nephropathy (Fischer rat)
8-Methoxypsoralen	Phototoxicity
Methyl mercury	Encephalopathy
Morphine	Physical & psychological dependence
MPTP	Parkinsonism
Musk ambrette	Photosensitivity
2-Naphthylamine	Bladder cancer (dog)
Neuroleptic drugs	Galactorrhoea
Nitrofurantoin	Testicular damage
Paraquat	Lung damage and fibrosis
Phenformin	Lactic acidosis
Phenothiazine NP 207	Retinopathy (pigmented animals)
Penicillamine	Loss of taste
Pyridoxin	Sensory neuropathy
Scopolamine	Behavioural disturbances
Slow release potassium	Intestinal ulceration
Thalidomide, prenatal	Phocomelia (monkey, rabbit)
Triorthocresylphosphate	Delayed neuropathy
Triparanol	Cataract
Vinyl chloride	Angiosarcoma of the liver
Vitamin A	Osteopathy
Vitamin D	Nephrocalcinosis

Expectations

What are our expectations from animal toxicity studies? The toxicity of the compound should be adequately characterised in several animal species, such that the clinician can be alerted to possible similar effects in man. A margin of safety over the proposed clinically effective dose should be established.

Since the effects of medicines are known to vary in the highly heterogenous human population by race, age, sex, physical and nutritional condition and disease state, it is not certain that the normal series of pharmacology or toxicology studies in healthy laboratory animals can be fully predictive. Subjective effects experienced by humans that are poorly predicted in animal tests include headache, dizziness, tinnitus, and vision disturbances. Skin rash and other immunotoxic effects are also difficult to predict; deWeck[2] in 1983 reported that hypersensitivity has been by far the most common drug induced immunopathy in man, accounting for 15 percent of the total untoward reactions to xenobiotics.

In attempting to evaluate drug safety from animal studies and the possible extrapolation of the results to humans, it is important to first define the objectives of the animal tests, the rationale for the study design, and the relationship of the animal dosing to the proposed clinical regimen. The acceptability of adverse side-effects of a new drug will depend on its proposed use. It is possible that some toxic effects would not be acceptable for the treatment of a relatively minor condition or one for which other drugs of greater safety already exist.

Toxicity studies

The toxicity studies, including single and multiple doses to animals, should initially support the careful administration of small doses to healthy human subjects (Phase I). Once the suitability of the animal species and the doses selected have been supported by comparison with absorption and pharmacokinetic data in man, the longer term toxicology studies can be designed to support the proposed clinical regimen for patients.

A most important aspect of the correlation of toxic effects is the selection of animal species in which the drug is absorbed, distributed, metabolised and excreted in a similar manner to man. The value of multi-species toxicity studies and parallel metabolic studies can be seen in studies with the synthetic cannabinoid and anti-emetic compound nabilone by Hanasono[3] et al. (1987). Daily oral dosing to rats, dogs and rhesus monkeys for ninety days did not produce significant toxic effects or pathological changes. Non dose-related cumulative toxicity was, however, observed in a one-year chronic study in dogs (top dose 2.0 mg/kg/day). The toxicity in dogs was attributed to the formation of carbinol metabolites that accumulated in the brain. These carbinol metabolites, formed by stereospecific enzymatic reduction of the 9-keto group of nabilone, were major metabolites in dogs but minor metabolites in rhesus monkeys and humans. The most realistic toxicological support for repeated dosing in humans was, therefore, provided by a subsequent one-year chronic toxicity study performed in rhesus monkeys in which no significant toxic effects were observed.

Mutagenicity and carcinogenicity

In considering expectations from studies, I would like to concentrate on two of the more difficult questions for the industrial toxicologist, namely, are mutagenicity and carcinogenicity tests predictive of potential carcinogenicity in humans?

For many years, potential new drugs have been tested at high doses in long-term carcinogenicity studies in rodents prior to regulatory approval and broad clinical use. These studies have been costly in test chemical, animals, laboratory facilities and staff, and research time. Although the overall database on animal bioassays has been greatly expanded by the testing of more than 300 chemicals in rodents by the United States National Cancer Institute and the National

Toxicology Programme, the prediction of human carcinogenicity is still problematic. In many studies, the results have varied between species, strains and the sexes of the animals tested. The incidence of tumours observed has not always been dose-related and the long debate by experienced pathologists and oncologists regarding the definition of benign and malignant lesions in rodents and their relevance to human carcinogenesis continues.

Since short-term mutagenicity tests are expected to detect genotoxic carcinogens, a strong rationale has been developed for the use of these tests early in the process of drug development. Initial data from short-term assays using bacteria, which claimed a good correlation between positive genotoxicity and carcinogenic effects in long-term animal studies, produced a proliferation of mutagenicity testing in the pharmaceutical industry and requirements for such data by regulatory agencies prior to the approval of new drugs. Although neither a positive nor a negative result in the short-term tests can be considered fully definitive, the International Agency for Research on Cancer[4] has noted that the majority of chemicals that have given sufficient evidence of inducing human tumours are genotoxic.

During recent years, it has become evident that the early estimates of the predictability of the mutagenicity tests for the carcinogenic properties of most chemicals was too optimistic[5,6]. A careful validation of *in vitro* tests against the results of long-term rodent carcinogenicity studies by Tennant *et al.*[6], found that none of the short-term tests were necessarily predictive. In fact, it was suggested that no combination of the mutagenicity tests was significantly better than a single test. Furthermore, Clayson[7] has suggested that short-term tests cannot be expected to detect all types of carcinogens since mutations may be only related to the initiation phase of the complex process of carcinogenesis.

In the toxicology research laboratories of Eli Lilly and Company, many compounds have been tested in several of the broadly used and well-accepted mutagenicity tests (Table 2).

In these validation studies, most of the known human or

animal carcinogens could be detected and only a few false-positives were observed (Table 3).

When research compounds were tested in this tier, the number of positive findings was relatively small and in no case has a compound produced a positive response in more than one test.

Table 2. Genetic toxicology test battery

In vitro tests
    Ames bacterial mutation
    L5178Y mammalian mutation
    Rat hepatocyte DNA repair
    Cho cell cytogenetics
In vivo tests
    Bone marrow cytogenetics
    Mouse micronucleus
    Rat hepatocyte DNA repair

Under these circumstances, we have considered there to be insufficient reason to prevent the continued development of the compound and subsequent administration to humans. In many cases, following a detailed review of the data, the compounds were progressed to long-term rodent studies and reproduction studies to ensure that no adverse effects were produced on somatic or germinal cells.

Table 3. Genetic toxicology data base, Eli Lilly & Company

Test System	Total	Validation studies Expected positives	Unexpected positives
Bacterial mutation	24	11	1
DNA repair	251	86	6
L5178Y mutation	71	38	4
In vitro cytogenetics	8	5	0
In vivo SCE	59	24	1
Mouse micronucleus	13	9	0

Design of studies

The acceptance of long-term rodent studies in assessing possible carcinogenic properties of new drugs is evidenced by their inclusion in the development programme of drugs for chronic dosing in humans and the requirements of the majority of world-wide regulatory agencies. The widely accepted study design involves the use of 50 to 60 animals per sex per dosage group at three dose levels plus one or two control groups. However, there are several issues relating to this design.

1. Although it is recognised that very large test groups of animals are needed to statistically demonstrate a low incidence of a carcinogenic effect, the use of such numbers is impractical in drug development. It has been argued that the use of "maximum tolerated doses" of the test compounds improves the statistical power of the tests to detect carcinogenic effects.
2. The hotly debated use of "maximum tolerated doses", which are often very large multiples of the proposed human dose, may certainly ensure exposure of the test compound and its metabolites, but may also overwhelm the metabolic capacity of the animals. The knowledge that a wide variety of drugs and other chemicals, in high doses, can induce, promote or modulate the occurrence of tumors in long-term rodent studies is a major complicating and concerning factor.
3. The problems in assessing human risk also assumes that the potency of a carcinogen is similar in the rodent species and humans and that the carcinogenic response will be observed above the high and variable incidence of the spontaneous tumors that occur in the given strain of animals employed. Examples of the most common incidence of tumor types by target organ in rodent carcinogenicity studies have been reported for many industrial toxicology laboratories in the United States in a Pharmaceutical Manufacturers Association Drug Safety Subsection Report[8]. This analysis has reported that liver and

mammary tumors were the most prevalent tumor types in rats whereas liver and pulmonary tumors were most prevalent in mice.

The recognition of the existence of non-genotoxic carcinogens, some of which possess hormonal properties and have produced tumors in reproductive organs in rodents, such as the thiourea thyroid carcinogens and some estradiol derivatives, together with compounds which may induce cancer by inducing hepatic hyperplasia and/or peroxisomal proliferation,[9] has supported the need for both mutagenic and long-term carcinogenic studies. Examples of drugs which have produced oncogenic effects in long-term studies due to exaggerated pharmacodynamic effects have been reported by Hottendorf[10].

Since most of the compounds that have progressed to long-term animal studies in our laboratories have given negative responses in mutagenicity studies and have not produced proliferative changes in subchronic toxicity studies, we have felt it important to analyse our historical data base consisting of nearly 70 long-term studies in rats and mice (Table 4). The rodents have usually been obtained from the same animal supplier and have been maintained under similar rodent diets *ad libitum*. The animals have been examined at necropsy by pathologists who also examined the tissues microscopically using widely accepted diagnostic criteria. The majority of the compounds tested have given negative results for carcinogenic effects.

Of the 20 studies which have given rise to scientific or regulatory problems, the data precluded the further development of the test compounds in only three cases. In each case the decision was based on a compound-related increased incidence of liver tumors. Following a detailed review of the other 17 cases, the responses were considered to be due to either exaggeration of the pharmacological properties of the compounds, physico-chemical effects such as irritation in the kidneys due to deposition of insoluble compounds from high doses, or marked induction of liver enzyme systems resulting in hepatic hyperplasia.

Table 4. Results of two-year carcinogenic studies
Eli Lilly and Company (1973–1988)

		Proportion of total studies		
Species/ strain	Number completed	With scientific and/or regulatory problems	Results precluded further development	No major effects observed
Wistar rat	14	4 (29%)	1	10
Fischer 344 rat	23	5 (22%)	0	18
ICR mouse	7	3 (43%)	1	4
B6C3F1 mouse	24	8 (33%)	1	16

Conclusion

We have concluded that the absence of a carcinogenic response in long-term rodent studies can provide a significant measure of confidence to proceed with the development of a new drug for chronic therapy in humans. I can therefore agree with the overall summary of Ashby and Tennant[11] who suggested that the detection of potential carcinogens can be best implemented by a comparison of the structure with similar compounds previously tested, a series of genotoxicity tests and carcinogenesis bioassays in rodents.

In summary, it is the responsibility of the toxicologist to design and conduct a series of comprehensive and defensible tests in animals to determine if potential new drugs are likely to be hazardous when used in human therapy. The extent and duration of the animal studies depends upon the scope of the clinical trials planned and the future therapeutic indication for the drug. The low proportion of significant toxic reactions in humans with new drugs compared to the total number tested and introduced, supports the contention that toxicity studies in laboratory animals are, in the main, predictive for humans.

References

1. Zbinden, G. (1985). *Menschen, Tiere und Chemie*, MTC Verlag, Zollikon, Switzerland.
2. deWeck, A.L. (1983). Immunopathological mechanisms and clinical aspects of allergic reactions to drugs. In: *Handbook of Experimental Pharmacology*, Vol 63. Allergic Reactions to Drugs. A.L. deWeck and H. Bundgaard (eds.) Springer-Verlag, New York, pp. 75–133.
3. Hanasono, G.K., Sullivan, H.R., Gries, C.L. Jordan, W.H. and Emmerson, J.L. (1987). A species comparison of the toxicity of Nabilone, a new synthetic cannabinoid. *Fund. Appl. Pharmacol.*, **9**: 185–197.
4. International Agency for Research on Cancer (1987). IARC Monographs on the evaluation of carcinogenic risks to humans, Suppl. 7, Over all evaluations of carcinogenicity: An updating of IARC monographs, Vols, 1–42, Lyon, France.
5. Shelby M.D. and Stasiewicz, S. (1984). Chemicals showing no evidence of carcinogenicity in long-term two species rodent studies; the need for short-term test data. *Environ. Mutagen.*, **6**: 871–876.
6. Tennant R.W., Margolin B.H., Shelby M.D., Zeiger E., Haseman J.K., Spalding J., Caspary W., Resnick M., Stasiewicz S., Anderson B. and Minor R. (1987). Prediction of chemical carcinogenicity in rodents from in vitro genetic toxicity assays. *Science*, **236**: 933–941.
7. Clayson, D.B. (1987). The need for biological risk assessment in reaching decisions about carcinogens. *Mutation Res.*, **185**: 243–269.
8. PMA (1989). Results of a questionnaire involving the design of and experience with carcinogenicity studies. (September, 1988) *U.S.P.M.A. Drug Safety Subsection*.
9. Butterworth B.E., Bermudez E., Smith Oliver T., Earle L., Cattley R., Martin J., Popp J.A., Strom S., Jirtle R. and Michalopoulos A. (1984). Lack of genotoxic activity of di(2-ethylhexyl)phthalate (DEHP) in rat and human hepatocytes. *Carcinogenesis*, **5**: 1329–1335.
10. Hottendorf, G.H. (1987). Progress in Drug Research, Vol. 31, 1987.
11. Ashby J. and Tennant R.W. (1988). Chemical structure, Salmonella mutagenicity and extent of carcinogenicity as indices of genotoxic carcinogens among 222 chemicals tested in rodents by the U.S. NCI/NTP. *Mutation Res.*, **204**: 17–115.

2
The importance of retrospective comparisons

ROGER BRIMBLECOMBE

Summary

1. Prospective studies designed to assess the relevance of animal toxicity studies for man are rarely possible for ethical reasons.
2. Retrospective collection and analysis of data represent less satisfactory, but important, alternatives.
3. Such data are available within single organisations especially pharmaceutical companies, but analysis of larger data bases, e.g. those in regulatory agencies or collected (by, for example, the Centre for Medicines Research) from a number of companies, has the potential for yielding more valuable information.
4. A retrospective study carried out within Smith Kline & French is described and its limitations, value and conclusions discussed.
5. A major conclusion from the study is that collation of internal data with those from outside sources to provide a larger relevant data base has been shown to be valuable on several occasions.

Introduction

Discussions concerning the relevance and predictive value for man of animal toxicity studies are limited by a paucity of data. Substances showing marked toxicity in animals can only rarely, for ethical reasons, be administered to man. Prospective studies are, therefore, only possible with substances showing an acceptable toxicological profile in animals. Retrospective analyses, while less satisfactory, still represent valuable sources of information.

Retrospective studies can take a number of forms:

1. Re-evaluation of data from animal studies when unwanted effects occur subsequently and unexpectedly in man.
2. Design of specific animal studies to elucidate mechanisms of unwanted effects which have been observed in man.
3. Pooling of data from a number of sources to increase the size of the data base and to enable more meaningful "epidemiological-type" analyses to be performed.
4. Reviews of the history of individual compounds which have been, or are in, development.

Survey

A survey within Smith Kline & French Laboratories R & D revealed that between 1958 and 1987, 17 compounds were withdrawn from development (either preclinical or clinical) because of adverse findings in animal toxicity studies. Such findings contributed to the cessation of development of many more compounds but they were not judged to be the sole or the main reason and so these compounds were not included in the analysis.

It was concluded that in 4 of the 17 cases the decision to terminate the project might possibly be different in the light of current knowledge. In every case this was based on a better understanding of the lesion involved compared to when the study was originally evaluated. These lesions included carcinoid tumours of the rat gastric mucosa (long-acting antisecretory agent), myocardial lesions affecting the papillary muscle of dogs (inotropic agents) and mesenteric arteritis in rats (dopamine-like compounds).

Amongst the other 13 compounds it was considered that the decision to discontinue development would be no different today because one or more of the factors shown in Table 1 applied.

Table 1. Factors confirming the decision to terminate development

1. No, or very low, ratio between the dose producing significant toxicity in animals and the anticipated human therapeutic dose.
2. Lack of understanding of the mechanism of toxicity or its relevance to man.
3. Clear indication that the lesion *has* relevance for man.

Also considered in this review were compounds which were still in development following satisfactory explanation of potentially serious toxicological findings in animals. These are shown in Table 2.

Table 2. Compounds still in development

Carcinoid tumours in rats with a potent antisecretory agent. This is now generally accepted to be a sequel of hypergastrinaemia and probably of little relevance in the therapeutic use of such compounds in man.

Mesenteric arteritis in rats (but not dogs or monkeys) with a dopamine agonist. Investigations showed that this apparently rat specific, lesion was also seen with dopamine.[1]

Cardiac arteritis in beagles (but not other species). Consultation with other companies and, eventually, a Toxicology Forum[2] meeting revealed that the lesion was more commonly seen than had been thought. Its toxicological significance for man was considered to be low[3].

Conclusion

Conclusions drawn from this study are:

(i) This, and similar studies, even if they are on a larger scale, do not enable definitive conclusions to be drawn concerning the predictiveness for man of serious toxic effects seen in animals especially when the dose and/or the mechanism of the effect is not understood - such substances are not administered to man.
(ii) The value of investigative studies to gain further understanding of toxic effects is demonstrated. Three compounds proceeded in development despite significant toxicity in animals. One compound (producing haemolysis *in vivo* in animal studies subsequently proved to be haemolytic *in vitro* in other species including man) was immediately withdrawn from development.
(iii) It is essential to put the toxicological findings into context against an ever-changing knowledge base. This base must be expanded and kept up-to-date from whatever sources are available – internal, open literature, but especially from other similar organisations with similar problems.

In contrast to the situation where compounds showing appreciable toxicity in animals are rarely administered to man, there are very large numbers of examples of substances which have not shown marked toxicity in animals being given to man. This fact, in itself, displays confidence in the predictive value of animal studies and, although precise data are hard to come by, this confidence seems to be born out in practice. Only rarely have unsuspected adverse effects been seen in man although these inevitably receive more publicity than the majority of cases. Often such compounds display hypersensitivity reactions or produce essentially subjective side-effects for both of which animal studies are of limited value.[4]

References

1. Kerns, W.D., Arena.A., Macia, R.A., Bugelski, P.J., Matthews, W. D. and Morgan, D.G. (1989). Pathogenesis of arterial lesions induced by dopaminergic compounds in the rat. *Toxicologic Pathology*, **17**: 203–213.
2. *Toxicologic Pathology*, **17** (1) (Pt 2), 1989.
3. Issacs, K.R., Joseph, E.C. and Betton, G.R. (1989). Coronary vascular lesions in dogs treated with phosphodiesterase III inhibitors. *Toxicologic Pathology*, **17**: 153–163.
4. Griffin, J.P. (1986). Predictive value of animal toxicity studies. In *Long-Term Animal Studies – Their Predictive Value for Man.* ed Walker S.R. and Dayan A.D., MTP Press, Lancaster, England, pp. 107–117.

II. Methodology: A Critical Approach

A. The Global Approach

3
Antineoplastics, a unique group

PHILIP SCHEIN

Summary

1. The field of oncology is in a unique position to enable retrospective or prospective analyses of the predictive validity of animal testing and to determine to what extent these data are of practical value for avoiding serious adverse reactions.
2. Published studies show that the introduction of a new anticancer agent at one-tenth to one-third the maximum tolerated dose of the more sensitive animal species provides a safe method for initiating a Phase I clinical trial.
3. For 25 anti-cancer agents, a retrospective analysis of dog and monkey predictions of human organ system toxicity has shown that correct predictions are accomplished at the cost of a high percentage of false positives, particularly for renal and hepatic toxicity.
4. There is a need for further research in the field of drug safety evaluation, including a further refinement of the current understanding of the relative sensitivity of specific organs to toxic effects in each of the relevant species.

Introduction

The role of animal toxicology as a predictive system for drug toxicity in man is particularly relevant to the field of cancer chemotherapy[1,2]. Anticancer agents, as a group, fail in varying degrees to discriminate efficiently between normal and target issues. A wide range of qualitative toxicities are both anticipated and encountered, and with many drugs the administration of moderately toxic doses is regarded as a requirement in order to achieve a therapeutic response. An additional factor relates to the nature of the patient population, a proportion of which are already debilitated by the disease process or previous therapy, and therefore are potentially less tolerant of drug toxicity. The principal objective of animal toxicology is to generate information about the new agent that will forewarn the physician about potential drug hazards that may be encountered during the initial clinical trial. In the process, toxicity data are necessarily extrapolated from one species to another, with the implicit assumption that data derived from specific animal species have predictive value for man and that important toxicity will not go unpredicted.

Over the years many protocols have evolved, which in some cases go beyond the simple purpose of the safe introduction of a new agent. The validity or justification of each phase of a programme of toxicity testing has rarely been questioned. Specifically, which studies provide practical guidelines for the safe introduction of a new compound in man, and which aspects represent "research" to advance the science of drug safety evaluation? Additionally, what is the cost/benefit of extensive animal testing in terms of budget, animals sacrificed and time frames which may unnecessarily delay the introduction of a drug into clinical practice?

The field of oncology is in a unique position to define an efficient system of toxicology evaluation in preparation for Phase I clinical trials. Anticancer drugs are particularly toxic, with emphasis on rapidly dividing tissues such as the bone marrow, gastrointestinal epithelium and organs of fertility. A relatively high incidence of toxic reactions are observed in all species. It is therefore possible to prepare retrospective or prospective analyses of the predictive validity of animal testing to determine to what extent these data are of practical value for avoiding serious adverse reactions.

Determination of a safe starting dose for phase I clinical trial

Freireich et al. examined the ability of six animal species to predict the maximum tolerated dose (MTD) of anticancer agents[3]. This analysis demonstrated that mouse, rat, dog, monkey and man have essentially the same maximum tolerated dose when data are compared on mg/sq m of body surface area. The results of the study support the initiation of Phase I clinical trials at a dose that is one-third that of an animal MTD. The mouse proved to be as useful as any other species in this regard. This study was followed by a similar review performed by Homan who applied a regression analysis to the MTD's of twenty-five anticancer drugs that had been tested in dog and monkey[4]. It was estimated that a dose 1/10 of the dog MTD in mg/sq m carried a 1.3% risk of exceeding the human MTD in Phase I testing, whereas the corresponding risk for monkey data was 1.1%. If the initial clinical dose was increased to 1/3 the mg/sq m animal MTD, the risk for exceeding the human MTD was 10% for each of the animal species, and 6% if the more sensitive species was used.

A further study was performed by Goldsmith et al.[5] in which a retrospective analysis of the ability of mouse, dog and monkey to predict for the quantitative toxicity of 30 anticancer agents was undertaken. The mouse proved to be as useful, if not a better predictive model, as the dog and monkey, for insuring a safe starting dose for man. Using 1/3 the mg/sq m of the LD_{10} of normal mice, this species overpredicted the human MTD for only two of twenty-nine drugs tested. The corresponding dose in dogs and monkeys would have resulted in 21–24% of the initial doses in man to have been toxic. Rozencweig et al.[6] conducted an analysis of twenty-one anticancer agents in which murine and dog data were compared to human, using identical schedules of administration. These investigators found that 1/6 the LD_{10} in the mouse or 1/3 the toxic dose low (TDL) in the dog correspond to acceptable starting doses in man. The authors concluded that the starting dose in Phase I clinical trials could be safely and efficiently based on $1/10$ LD_{10} in the mouse, with prior verification that this dose was not lethal or life threatening in the dog as an added safety measure.

The results of each of these studies are similar; the introduction of a new anticancer drug at 1/10 to 1/3 the MTD of the more sensitive animal species provides a safe method for initiating a Phase I clinical trial. In general, data derived from murine studies are at least as informative as that obtained from dogs and monkeys. As a result, mouse toxicology studies have increasingly become a principal determinant for estimating initial doses to be used in humans. Guarino *et al.*[7] have, however, cautioned that several parameters may modify the toxicity of anticancer agents in mice, in particular strain, drug vehicle and route of administration.

Prediction of qualitative toxicities

A detailed retrospective analysis of dog and monkey predictions of human organ system toxicity has been reported for twenty-five anticancer agents of diverse chemical and functional classification[8]. This study utilised data that were accrued from the NCI Toxicology Programme that required both the determination of acute lethal toxicity in dogs as well as subacute toxicology in dogs and monkeys[9]. Approximately 170 parameters of toxicity were analysed using this large computer data base.

The dog and monkey proved to be equivalent in their prediction of leukopenia with 60 and 61% true-positive and 20 and 17% false-negatives, respectively (Table 1). An important and novel aspect of the data base, at the time, was the demonstration that the monkey is quite resistant to the development of thrombocytopenia; this species produced 56% false-negative predictions compared to 19% for the dog. In the case of gastrointestinal toxicity, the dog once again proved to be the superior predictive species with 92% true-positive and no false-negatives compared to 74% true-positive and 14% false-negatives for the monkey (Table 2). The monkey proved to be quite resistant to the emetogenic properties of anticancer agents. Both species grossly overpredicted for hepatic toxicity with 44% false-positives for the dog and 35% for the monkey. A similar overprediction was noted for the estimation of renal toxicity: the dog produced a 56% false-positive index and 20% false- negatives, whereas the monkey produced 48% false-positives and 10% false-negatives.

Table 1. Prediction of haematologic toxicity

	TP* %	FP %	TN %	FN %	FN / TP+FN %	Number of Compounds Tested
Anaemia						
Dogs	44	28	24	4	8	25
Monkeys	35	43	9	13	27	23
Dogs & Monkeys	48	44	8	0	0	25
Leukopenia						
Dogs	60	4	16	20	25	25
Monkeys	61	13	9	17	22	23
Dogs & Monkeys	68	12	8	12	15	25
Thrombocytopenia						
Dogs	59	14	14	13	19	22
Monkeys	32	0	27	41	56	22
Dogs & Monkeys	54	12	13	21	28	24
Haematologic Toxicity						
Dogs	80	12	0	8	9	25
Monkeys	83	13	0	4	5	23
Dogs & Monkeys	88	12	0	0	0	25

*TP=True positive
FP=False positive
TN=True negative
FN=False negative
FN/TP+FN=Corrected false negative, which analyses the predictions for only those compounds that produced the specific toxicity in man.

This analysis was followed by the study reported by Rozencweig et al.[6] in which qualitative toxicities reported for mice and dogs were compared with those in man. The predictive value of organ system toxicity in animals was found to depend on the prevalence of this toxicity in the human species.

Table 2. Prediction of gastrointestinal toxicity

	TP* %	FP %	TN %	FN %	FN/TP+FN %	Number of Compounds Tested
Vomiting						
Dogs	72	16	0	12	14	25
Monkeys	26	13	4	57	68	23
Dogs & Monkeys	72	16	0	12	14	25
Diarrhoea						
Dogs	36	40	20	4	10	25
Monkeys	13	26	35	26	66	23
Dogs & Monkeys	36	44	16	4	10	25
Gastrointestinal Toxicity						
Dogs	92	8	0	0	0	25
Monkeys	74	9	0	17	19	23
Dogs & Monkeys	92	8	0	0	0	25

*TP=True positive
FP=False positive
TN=True negative
FN=False negative
FN/TP+FN=Corrected false negative, which analyses the predictions for only those compounds that produced the specific toxicity in man.

Positive predictions were highest for commonly observed adverse reactions in man, such as gastrointestinal intolerance and myelosuppression. However, positive predictions declined dramatically with rare toxic manifestations. There was no clear superiority of animal findings over the knowledge of the prevalence of these toxicities in humans. The authors concluded that the routine and undiscerned investigation of organ system toxicity in animals is of questionable usefulness for clinical trials with chemotherapeutic agents.

Conclusion

Useful data relating to a safe initial clinical dose can be derived from studies in either mice or dogs. This is the essential first step in any Phase I clinical trial, since once the safety of the initial dose has been demonstrated, the drug can be carefully escalated to a maximum tolerated dose or effective schedule. There appears to be no reason to conduct these studies in monkeys since this species does not offer an advantage over rodents and dogs. Data relating to qualitative organ system toxicities, to the extent they provide useful information, can be defined in dogs and perhaps rodents in acute and subacute studies. The latter is important to insure that toxicities requiring a cumulative injury for expression might be demonstrated, as well as to furnish additional data for multiple dose clinical trials. Typically Phase I trials of anticancer agents utilise single dose and daily-times-five schedules which are further expanded based upon results of the initial experience. Once again, monkey data did not significantly add to the prediction of qualitative toxicities in man.

Correct predictions of organ toxicity are accomplished at the cost of a high percentage of false-positives; this is particularly the case for renal and hepatic toxicity. Several possible explanations for the high incidence of overprediction can be offered. In order to elicit all qualitative toxicities inherent in a new drug, animals are routinely given severely toxic and sometimes lethal dose levels. This stands in contrast to Phase I clinical trials where typically a study is discontinued when the first dose-limiting toxicity is encountered. There does appear, however, to be definite differences in species- related organ system sensitivity to drug toxicity. Toxicity to a human organ may be expressed in a different specific clinical or chemical parameter, or at a lesser or greater dose than in the animal. In addition, the adverse reaction may take a different order of appearance in relationship to the total spectrum of qualitative toxicities inherent in the new drug. The animals do, however, identify a high percentage of drugs that produce some of the more commonly experienced toxicities associated with cancer chemotherapy, such as bone marrow suppression. The animal toxicology screen has, in general, correctly identified drugs which are less toxic to the bone marrow, such as bleomycin and streptozotocin. This is a particularly important feature for a new antineoplastic in view of the recognised myelosuppresive properties of most available chemotherapeutic agents. Lastly, the animal screen has on occasion predicted those drugs in which toxicity was delayed in onset; this was demonstrated in the case of the chloroethylnitrosureas, although the predictions did not directly correlate with the organ system affected in man.

In 1979, the FDA Oncology Drugs Advisory Committee reviewed this information and made recommendations to simplify the toxicology requirements for Phase I studies of new antineoplastic agents. These recommendations were adopted by the National Cancer Institute. A new protocol for toxicological testing was initiated which called for acute dose-ranging studies in mice in order to estimate the starting clinical dose, as well as acute studies in dogs and mice to access the qualitative toxicities inherent in the new agent[10]. Each drug was to be administered as a single dose or on a five consecutive day schedule, with animals to be sacrificed in the acute toxicity studies at various points after dosing was completed. There was to be complete haematologic and clinical chemistry evaluations as well as pathology on each animal in the study. In 1983 rats were substituted for mice for the acute toxicity studies in rodents in order to provide a larger animal for blood collection for clinical laboratory assessment.

There remains a continued need for further research in the field of drug safety evaluation, including a further refinement of our current understanding of the relative sensitivity of specific organs to toxic effects in each of the relevant species. It must be recognised, however, that animals may fail to predict for many important toxicities subsequently discovered in man. There are many such examples in the field of oncology, including pancreatitis observed during clinical trials of L-asparaginase and anthracycline-induced cardiac toxicity, which were unappreciated in dogs and monkeys during the toxicology evaluations. These examples of underprediction by animals may represent inherent biological differences amongst the species, as is clearly demonstrated by the resistance of the monkey to the development of thrombocytopenia and gastrointestinal toxicity, two very prominent forms of adverse reactions in man. In some cases a false-negative may reflect the relatively small number of animals used in toxicity evaluation compared to the large number of patients who receive the new drug. In addition, normal, healthy animals are routinely employed in toxicology studies in contrast to the patient population with which they are being compared. The patients with cancer who are candidates for chemotherapy typically have advanced disease that may affect normal organ function, and in the case of individuals being placed in Phase I trials, they have in most instances received prior standard chemotherapy. Patients are almost always receiving concomitant medications, including antiemetics, analgesics and hypnotics, all which may complicate the interpretation of clinical data.

Ultimately, the initiation and conduct of a safe and informative Phase I clinical trial requires a realistic understanding of the limits of animal toxicology data coupled with careful monitoring, judgement and expectation by a trained and experienced clinical pharmacologist.

References

1. Glicksman, A.S. and Schein, P.S. (1985). Acute and late effect of cancer therapy in medical oncology. In *Basic Principles and Clinical Management of Cancer*, P. Calabresi, P.S. Schein and S.A. Rosenberg, (eds). pp 426–453, Macmillan, New York.
2. Schein, P.S. (1977). Preclinical toxicology of anticancer agents, *Cancer Res.*, **37**: 1934–1937.
3. Freireich, E.J., Gehan, E.A., Rall, D.P. Schmidt, L.H. and Skipper, H.E. (1966). Quantitative comparison of toxicity of anticancer agents in mouse, rat, hamster, dog, monkey and man, *Cancer Chemotherapy Rept.*, **50**: 219–244.
4. Homan, E.R. (1972). Quantitative relationships between toxic doses of antitumor chemotherapeutic agents in animals and man. *Cancer Chemotherapy Rept.* **3** (Part 3): 13–19.
5. Goldsmith, M.A., Slavik, M. and Carter, S.K. (1975). Quantitative prediction of drug toxicity in humans from toxicology in small and large animals. *Cancer Res.*, **35**: 1354–1364.
6. Rozencweig, M., Von Hoff, D.D., Staguet, M.J., Schein, P.S., Penta, J.S. et al., (1981). Animal toxicology for early clinical trials with anticancer agents. *Cancer Clin. Trials*, **4**: 21–28.

7. Guarino, A.M., Rozencweig, M. Kline, I., Penta, J.S., Venditi, J.M. *et al.*, Adequacies and inadequacies in assessing murine toxicity data with antineoplastic agents. *Cancer Res.*, **39**: 2204–2210.
8. Schein P.S., Davis, R.O., Carter, S.K., Newman, J., Schein, D.R. and Rall, D.P. (1970). The evaluation of anticancer drugs in dogs and monkeys for the prediction of qualitative toxicities in man. *Clin. Pharmacol. Ther.*, **14**: 3–40.
9. Cancer Chemotherapy National Service Centre (1964). An outline of procedures for preliminary toxicologic and pharmacologic evaluation of equipment cancer chemotherapeutic agents. *Cancer Chemotherapy Rept.*, **37**: 1–33.
10. Grieshaber, C.K. and Marsonl, S. (1986). Relation of preclinical toxicology to findings in early clinical trials. *Cancer Treat. Rept.*, **70**: 65–72.

4
What can be learnt by examining the data in the files of regulatory authorities? – the toxicologist's viewpoint

ROLF BASS

Summary

1. Data in the files of regulatory authorities highlight the problem areas that exist in extrapolating the results of animal studies to man.
2. Since animal toxicity studies should be performed for the sake of man, which implies differences for each developmental product, it is no longer appropriate to work to generalised and rigid guidelines.
3. The way in which regulatory authorities of European Community member states are trying to approach flexibility and interaction is described.
4. The question to be answered is not whether studies available retrospectively have been of relevance to man, but how to make such studies useful and relevant in the future.

Introduction

The availability of appropriate data before approving a drug for marketing has been made an ethical issue, the legal responsibility resting with the pharmaceutical manufacturer. Understandably, the same must also hold when administering developmental compounds to man.

Historically this has led from self-administration and self-observation of drugs and their effects, through the use of some animals that happened to be available at the time when interesting compounds were discovered, to the current situation where the non-usefulness of developmental compounds is judged from *l'art pour l'art* "battery" toxicological trials, referred to as scientific pre-clinical investigation. On the other hand, as soon as a positive decision has been made to continue development, new experimentation is necessary to disprove the relevance for man of toxic effects observed in the so-called animal models. Are regulatory authorities to believe that the results from the first type of animal toxicity studies constantly show serious signs of irrelevant toxicity and those from the second type always prove the absence of relevance? It can be easily learnt from the data in our files that this is not necessarily true, even if for the simple reason that positive data, once documented, cannot be wiped out by using negative ones as an eraser.

Problem areas

1. Observation of adverse events and adverse drug reactions in man but not in animals.
    It is possible that the effects in question either were not included in the battery test programme, were not noticed, or, although observed, were falsely interpreted. It is also possible that the effects in question may, according to the state of the art, not be observable and appropriate models may not be available.

    Retrospective analysis, case by case and generalising, can be addressed by those having full access to the files of pharmaceutical manufacturers. However, regulatory authorities have, I admit, played an important role in hindering investigators (or in making them feel hindered) to do this; proof is in our files.

2. Observation of adverse drug events in animals but not in man.

   The development and performance of current "safety" programmes unavoidably has led to overproduction of toxicity, concerning both the number of studies and the resultant effects. It is my duty to admit that regulatory authorities, representing public safety and opinion, have joined in a course allowing presentation of such cases at this meeting. Retrospective analysis, however, is easier than prospective exclusion of studies accepted to be unnecessary. How is one to deal with the valid statement that in case of doubt the error has to be placed on the safe side?

3. Adaption of toxicology programmes to the state of the art.

   When it comes to prospective guidance from scientific peers, proposals for changes of guidelines and test strategies seem as hard to come by from outside as from inside regulatory authorities. Guidance usually becomes available, helpful and supportive case, by case when reasonably trying to avoid extrapolation from animal toxicity to man or to specific conditions of use of a drug in man. From our files it becomes apparent that quite a few studies pinpointed now could have been prevented by more progressive guidelines; our business is a conservative one.

4. Problematic test areas.

   In most cases and countries it has been possible to prevent rigid guidelines from being enacted for those test areas where science has not supplied us yet with appropriate test systems or where good animal models are not available. This holds, for example, for the area of immune reactions. However, once the regulatory authority of one country has kindly asked for (inappropriate?) results to be submitted there seems to exist no escape clause; examples are on our files both ways.

The major area, where animal and experimental systems of refutable usefulness are available and required to be performed, is testing for oncogenic and carcinogenic potential. Their performance (or not) and their positive (and negative) outcome can be of substantial harm to the patient (and to the pharmaceutical manufacturer). We are all awaiting major changes to be put into our files so that superfluous long-term animal experimentation will no longer lead to results hardly to be explained to the public as being "in essence negative" or "irrelevant" for patients.

The area of sub-/chronic toxicity testing has been detested much less for the (in-) correctness of toxicity observed across species (including man) than for the inappropriateness of testing for too long. As soon as the scientific basis has been made available from the data bases of the pharmaceutical manufacturers (here I refer to the activities of the Centre for Medicines Research), legal changes for internationally introducing a "correct" time limit for chronic toxicity studies will have to be introduced. This is an example of a type of toxicity study where the problems have been recognised by all parties involved.

Other problem areas are those where human counterpart data practically do not exist, e.g. for the assessment of reproductive toxicity. Therefore, we can only learn from positive study results that they present us with a potential danger which may, case by case, prevent us from use leading to affected children or not. Since the introduction of current test systems no major drug catastrophe resulting from negative animal data has become evident. This is probably a main reason for the acceptance of the current situation, which can be found in the files of pharmaceutical manufacturers as well as those of regulatory authorities.

5. Reliable performance of toxicity studies.
   Here I would like to separate the formal GLP-requirements from the necessity for scientific conduct and evaluation. The farther away from the regulatory authority, the more stringent observation of GLP will be required; international acceptance of study data has increased everybody's demands. This is also the experience from our files. Obeyance of GLP-rules, however, will not be accepted as an excuse for bad scientific performance; this is also on file with us.

Case by case development

Since animal toxicity studies should be performed for the sake of man, which implies differences for each developmental product, the era of generally applicable and rigid guidelines must be declared over. Flexibility in itself seems insufficient, if the pharmaceutical manufacturer does not know how regulatory authorities will react to the test programmes envisioned, and if revision through interaction with the clinical level is not included.

The regulatory authorities of the member states of the EC are trying to approach flexibility and interaction, with their ideas being laid down in a draft "Note for Guidance on the Pre-Clinical Tests Required Prior to (and During) Clinical Trials". Since there exists no European harmonisation for clinical trials authorisation, pharmaceutical manufacturers should be put into a position allowing them to foresee what will be required across Europe. To gain access to regulatory authorities and to discuss with them the expected usefulness of the test programme and strategy laid down remains up to each pharmaceutical manufacturer insisting on his right to do so. To ask for programme changes and adaptations as the development goes on, requires reiteration of the same questions again and again; this will be requested by the regulatory authorities. Those studies which have not been requested until the end of clinical development, should not become necessary merely for registration purposes (with the exemption of ongoing oncogenicity–carcinogenicity studies).

To achieve all of these purposes the draft guideline avoids fixed correlations between pre-clinical and clinical test phases or stages and asks for detailed justification of programmes/strategies considering the state of the art in testing methods and procedures. For each broad class of toxicity testing guidance will be provided, firstly by asking about the type and extent of information available already (and thus possibly influencing programmes/strategies awaiting decision), secondly by asking to define the probability and then the suspicion in the test area, thirdly by relating to the duration and conditions of intended use in what type of patients, and finally, by deriving answers to these questions, reach a decision on the requirements of experimental studies in this class of toxicity testing and to be fed into the testing programme, thus yielding a reasoned strategy. As type, duration, and conditions of intended use as well as the type of patients may change as clinical trials proceed, each broad class of toxicity testing will have to be reviewed several times, taking into account the amount and type of knowledge accumulated, in man and animal, so far. Requirements for animal study programmes will, therefore, be guided by risk identification, evaluation of probabilities of risk and lead to practical steps of risk estimation for man. Depending on the degree of real suspicion of adverse effects to the expected, experimental clarification will have to be performed. The line of reasoning should be open to review and discussion with regulatory authorities which, thereby, can easily be put into a position of reasoned (dis-) agreement with the pharmaceutical manufacturer's (un) reasoned strategy.

Conclusion

When looking at one's data files the question to be answered is not whether the studies available retrospectively have been of relevance to man and to what extent or percentage, but how to make such studies useful and relevant in the future. This implies that in the past a number of investigations have yielded irrelevant results or were superfluous.

In order to increase the relevance of animal studies for the situation expected in man, early interaction between the pharmaceutical manufacturer and regulatory authorities may be needed case by case. If this interaction, based on the guidance described, leads to satisfactory results before, during and before the end of clinical trials, they should suffice also for registration purposes, exempting only certain groups, like orphan- or VIP-drugs. The proposed intertwining between pre-clinical and clinical investigations provides further guidance on the necessity and type of pre-clinical testing programmes. All these measures can be expected to reduce the overall number of toxicological studies, rendering those remaining as requirements more relevant.

5
What can be learnt by examining the data in the files of regulatory authorities? The clinician's viewpoint

PETER FLETCHER

Summary

1. A study was conducted in 1977 in which animal and clinical data for 45 compounds reviewed by the CSM were compared.
2. Problems concerning the regulatory authorities at that time are described and compared with current issues.
3. The files of regulatory authorities are unique in that they cover a whole range of compounds and therapeutic classes, together with the full spectrum of toxicological and clinical data.
4. An examination of this data could help to rationalise toxicity testing requirements, of which there has been a proliferation over the past decade.

Introduction

In 1977, when I was the Medical Assessor at the CSM, I wrote a paper[1] about the ways in which Regulatory Authority data could be used when examining the usefulness of animal toxicity tests. This presentation will be a retrospective look at what went on then and what has happened in the intervening period.

Regulatory Environment

The regulatory environment that existed at that time was much influenced by various demands that were being made on the authority. There were a number of matters that concerned the regulatory authority in the UK, for example Product Licences were taking between 12 and 24 months to approve. More importantly Clinical Trial Certificates (CTCs) were taking between 6 and 12 months, and sometimes even longer, and this was also of major concern to the pharmaceutical industry.

Professor David Grahame-Smith's working party actually developed from that discontent and its remit was to look at ways of shortening the review periods. At that time, full fertility testing was required before a CTC was granted, which essentially meant fairly long-term toxicity studies at that stage. This was one of the first things that the Grahame-Smith Working Party looked at, and subsequently this requirement was dropped. Recommendations on post-marketing surveillance were also made which were published a number of years later[2], so it was a long time in gestation.

Almost the whole of the Medicines Division's work at that time was related to new product applications and CTCs, with very few appeals (one a month or less). Professor Inman was making the first proposals for various post-marketing surveillance (PMS) systems and we were all becoming involved in the developing CPMP situation.

Dominating issues

At that time we were all dominated by two things: thalidomide and practolol. The practolol problem was just behind us and resulted in carcinogenicity testing becoming a requirement for CTCs for beta blockers. This cast a feeling of doom, despondency and despair in the minds of all the pharmaceutical companies because they saw their attempt to abbreviate pre-CTC requirements through the Grahame-Smith working party result in an even worse situation. It was a nasty shock that the practolol problem turned up; it was of course not predicted by animals and it took a long time to detect.

There were however quite a number of other things going on at that particular time, including clozepine agranulocytosis (a curious finding of clusters of patients in Finland alone), phenformin and lactic acidosis, and some curious toxicological findings with nalidixic acid (Charcot-like lesions in young animals) resulting in the decision that it should not be given to anyone under the age of 18. We were also beginning to receive reports from the United States and one of these was the possible carcinogenicity of spironolactone. There were various lipid lowering agents which were causing difficulty at the time, and one of them, tibric acid, also had reports of carcinogenicity associated with it. A rather unusual one, penfluridol, was a carcinogen of the pancreas, and then there was the saga of salbutamol induced mesovarian leiomyomas and their possible or impossible relevance to human beings.

It must be born in mind that in those days the Medicines Act was very much in its infancy. It had been instituted in 1972, so we were only three or four years into it, and beginning to learn its various powers and its deficiencies. These issues illustrate the fairly broad spectrum of material coming in to the regulatory authority at that time. Much of it was related to toxicity and a wealth of information was therefore available.

Retrospective study

The study I shall describe, involved 45 drugs which had been looked at virtually (but not entirely) consecutively by the Committee on Safety of Medicines (CSM) in the previous 12 to 18 months. All the relevant data were extracted from the files, and then all the animal studies including not only safety studies, but also physiological studies etc. were examined. Each adverse or toxicological effect occurring in an animal experiment was noted as one toxic effect. No refinements were made on this crude method, which was similar to collecting adverse events in that everything was included whether or not it was thought to be drug-associated. The clinical data was treated in the same way. For all the clinical trials, whether they were volunteer studies, phase II or phase III, all reported adverse events were noted. Animal and clinical effects were then compared with the aim of establishing correlations where they existed.

This study is still one of the very few that have made a direct comparison of findings in animal test systems and clinical trials on patients. A continuing problem is that it is only governmental agencies that have access to data generated for registration purposes on a full range of drugs seeking marketing approval. The study demonstrated that animal safety evaluation studies do have relevance in assessing positive clinical effects in patients, but that a considerable measure of uncertainty is involved. Certain effects seen in animals, such as vomiting, are highly correlated with the same effect in humans, whereas others, such as hypotension, are very poorly correlated.

Proliferation of guidelines

Since 1977 there has been an increase in the number of guidelines; the CPMP toxicology guidelines, the OECD toxicity testing guidelines which covered a whole range of chemicals, and the Annexes of the Sixth Amendment Directive of the EEC which were also toxicological guidelines. The Sixth Amendment concerned packaging and labelling directives which sought to classify certain substances as dangerous, toxic, mutagenic, teratogenic etc. The Directive applied mainly to industrial chemicals, pesticides, paint solvents and other non-pharmaceutical products. In addition there were Guidelines for Good Laboratory Practice. The result of this has been the development of a multiplicity of different guidelines which are similar but not identical. The problem is that it has codified and ritualised toxicity testing so that there is very little flexibility. In my view this is not ideal as we need a flexible system in which there is a possibility of matching toxicological requirements to particular compounds.

So where are we now? There are still toxicological problems and these have been dominated in recent years by the nonsteroidal anti-inflammatory agents, as practolol dominated in 1977. In addition the retinoids are now causing regulatory concern in many countries as they were in 1977. It was known that they were teratogenic from the start, but it has taken ten years for this to become a matter of public concern. The USA has taken a number of adequate steps to deal with these, but it illustrates that toxicological findings can take a long time to gain attention.

Conclusion

Whole animals are likely to remain the only realistic method of preclinical safety testing and more than a decade after this study not much has changed. There is a great deal of potential in examining the files of regulatory authorities as these have a unique value in that they cover a whole range of compounds and therapeutic classes, providing the full range of toxicological and clinical testing. Any one company will only have the information on its own compounds, and the only place in which the totality exists is in the regulatory authorities.

Now could the situation be improved? Firstly, the inclusion of toxicokinetics in current safety evaluation studies provides the opportunity to compare pharmacokinetics and metabolism in animals with man and could prevent inappropriate conclusions being drawn with regard to animal and human conditions. Secondly, there is an urgent need for closer co-operation between toxicologists, and clinicians in the pharmaceutical industry. Finally, further detailed analyses of toxicological and clinical data available from regulatory authorities should be carried out. This could be approached in several ways.

(i) Tabulate and analyse all the anatomical, physiological and toxicological findings for particular groups of compounds, such as chemically or therapeutically similar compounds. This would provide some idea as to whether they were consistent or inconsistent, and what could and could not be relied upon.

(ii) Analysis of time relationships. This is another parameter that is very difficult to study unless several different compounds can be compared. From this situations could be identified that have proved to be consistently unreliable and inappropriate or irrelevant. For example, with non-steroidal anti-inflammatory agents, fairly severe gastric bleeding occurs at very low dose levels – very often at the same dose level that would be used in man. As it is known that virtually all NSAID's cause this, is there anything to be gained from long-term tests in dogs? The answer is that from retrospective analyses, long-term studies in dogs could be considered irrelevant. Numerous similar situations could be cited where existing knowledge could help to determine the most appropriate package of safety evaluation studies. The problem still remains that access to data in Regulatory Authorities is strictly limited. It seems that pharmaceutical companies are unwilling to open their files on new products even though, in the long run, this could bring benefits in respect of developmental costs and safety evaluation.

References

1. Fletcher, A.P. (1978). Drug safety tests and subsequent clinical experience. *J. Roy. Soc. Med.*, **71**: 693–696.
2. Grahame-Smith Working Party recommendations.

B. Clinical Toxicity – Could it have been Predicted?

6
Clinical toxicity: could it have been predicted?
Pre-marketing experience

CYNDY LUMLEY

Summary

1. Eighteen pharmaceutical companies in the UK, Switzerland and the USA have provided information on the 29 compounds for which they terminated development between 1st January 1975 and 31st December 1986 due to clinical toxicity.
2. Almost one-half of the clinical effects causing termination (14) were effects that are difficult to identify in animal tests, including central nervous system (CNS) disturbances, blood dyscrasias or skin reactions/allergies and only 2 of these (both blood dyscrasias) were detected in animal tests.
3. Adverse effects on the liver were a major cause of termination (9 NCEs). In 4 cases hepatotoxicity was predicted or confirmed by animal tests whereas for 3 compounds it was not (data are not available for the remaining 2 compounds).
4. A small proportion of compounds tested in man are terminated due to clinical toxicity (less than 10%).

Introduction

New medicines are routinely evaluated for toxicity in a rodent and a non-rodent species based on the assumption that animals have significant predictive value for toxicity in man. Few studies have been published to provide a basis for this premiss, although many toxicologists have advocated a systematic comparison of data from animal and human tests. A study has therefore been initiated to collect information on pharmaceutical compounds for which development was terminated on the basis of clinical toxicity, and to compare this with findings in preclinical animal studies. This paper reports the results of the pilot study and is presented for a critical discussion of the methodology employed.

Methodology

Initially, pharmaceutical companies in Europe and the USA were asked to provide information on:

1. the number of new chemical entities (NCEs) for which they had made an application to conduct studies in patients, between 1st January 1975 and 31st December 1986;
2. the NCEs for which development was terminated on the basis of clinical toxicity, between 1st January 1975 and 31st December 1986, together with a description of the clinical effect causing termination.

Subsequently, all compounds identified in part 2 were followed up to ascertain whether any corresponding effects had been identified at any time during animal tests.

Results

Eighteen pharmaceutical companies in the UK, Switzerland and the USA took part in this study. Participating companies made an application to conduct clinical trials with 320 NCEs between 1st January 1975 and 31st December 1986, but information is not available to indicate the numbers tested in healthy volunteers. Over this time period, these companies terminated the development of 29 compounds on the basis of clinical toxicity (Table 1).

Table 1. Number of compounds terminated due to clinical toxicity

Number of compounds terminated	Number of companies
0	4
1	7
2	4
3	1
5	1
6	1

Although it is not possible to ascertain the exact proportion of compounds studied clinically that were terminated due to toxic effects in man, from the data collected it would appear that this is less than 10%. This confirms the findings of a study of NCEs evaluated by the 7 UK-owned companies[1] which also showed that 10% are terminated due to adverse effects in man (Figure 1).

The clinical toxicity causing termination of almost one-half (14) of the compounds (Table 2) was related to effects on the central nervous system, blood dyscrasias or skin reactions/allergies. It is widely accepted that these types of adverse reaction are difficult to identify in animal tests. Of the remaining 15 reactions, 5 were predicted or subsequently confirmed in animals, 5 were not predicted and for 5 further information is not available.

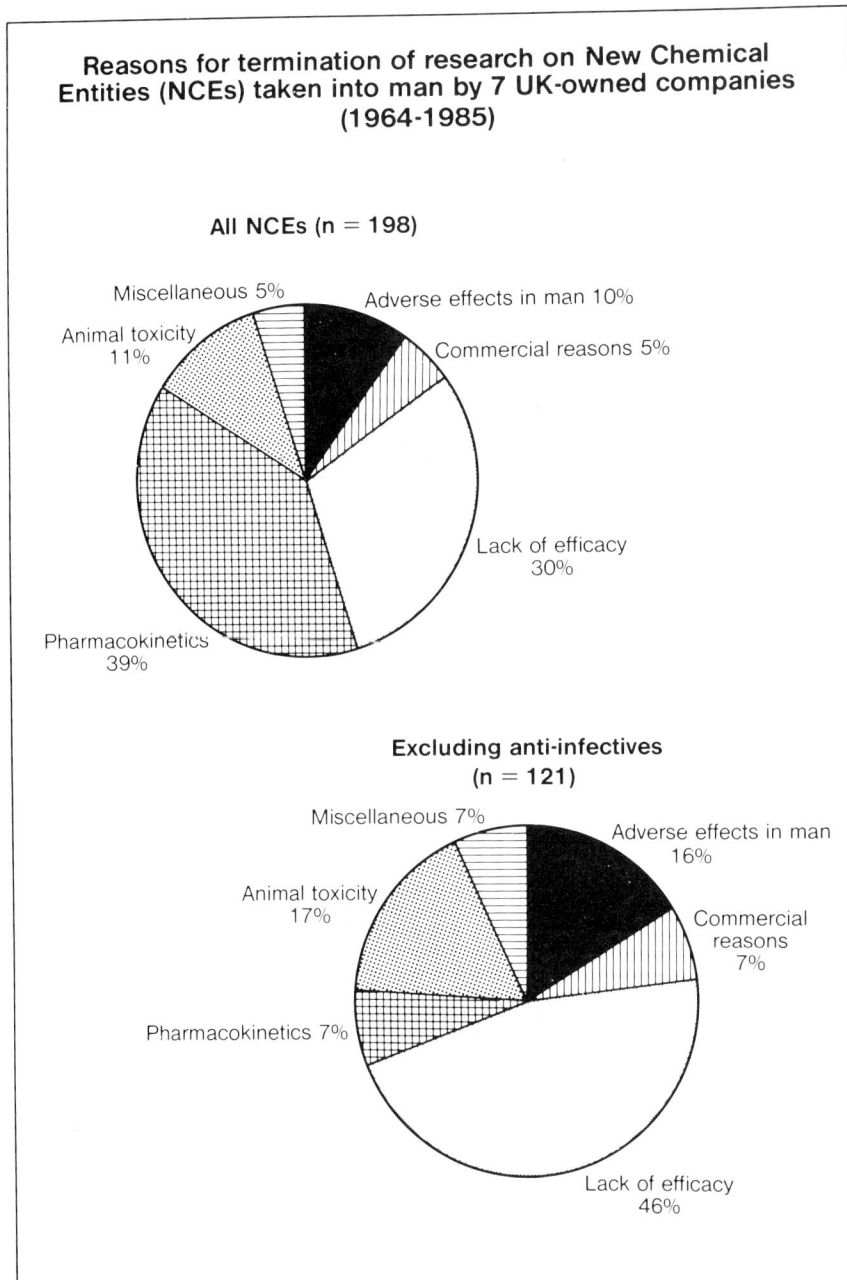

Figure 1 Reasons for termination of research

Table 2. compounds for which development was terminated on the basis of clinical toxicity

Therapeutic class	Phase of Testing	Approx. No./Vol. patients tested	Clinical toxicity	Predicted (Y/N) or confirmed (C) in animal tests
1. GI	Clin Trial	2000	Raised Liver Enzymes	C
2. CVS	n/a	n/a	Abnormal Liver Function Tests	n/a
3. CVS	Post-market		Hepatic Necrosis	N
4. CVS	Phase I/II		Increased transaminases	Y
5. Respiratory	n/a	n/a	Abnormal Liver Function Tests	n/a
6. NSAID	Phase III	2000	Raised Liver Enzymes	N
7.	Clin Trial	n/a	Raised Liver Enzymes	N
8. Antiallergy	Clin Trial	100s	Hepatoxicity	C
9. Antisecretory	Volunteers		Liver Abnormalities	Y
10. CVS	Volunteers	3	Rashes	N
11. Skin	Phase II	150	Skin reactions	N
12. PG inhibitor	n/a	n/a	Topical reaction	n/a
13. Spermicide	Volunteers	<10	Local irritability	N
14. Antiinfect	Volunteers		Pain on Injection	N
15. Endocrine	Phase II	35	Allergy	N*
16. CNS	Phase II	14	Allergy	N
17. n/a	Volunteers		Anaphylactic reaction	N
18. GI	Volunteers	10s	Tachycardia	N
19.	Phase II	60	Postural hypotension	Y**
20. Antiallergy	Volunteers	10s	Flushing	N
21. GI	Clin Trial	100s	Granulocytopenia	C
22. Thrombolytic	Volunteers	10s	Haemorrhage	Y
23. n/a	Phase II	2-300	Blood dyscrasias	N
24. CNS	Volunteers	40	White cell count decreased	N
25. GI	Volunteers		CNS disturbances	N
26. CNS	Phase II	40	CNS effects	N
27. Steroid	Volunteers	10	Adrenal suppression	C
28. LTD-4 antagonist	n/a	n/a	GI effects (High Dose)	n/a
29. Antiinfective	n/a	n/a	n/a	n/a

*Partially expected from chemical structure
**Nausea/vomiting which would have limited clinical use was also observed
n/a Not available

Effects on the liver were a major cause of termination (9 NCEs). Eight of these were raised liver enzymes or abnormal liver function tests, and five occurred between 1983 and 1985, at a time when there was increased sensitivity to liver problems due to the publicity given to effects related to Benoxaprofen.

Hepatotoxicity was indicated in the animal studies for two of the nine compounds and subsequently confirmed in animals for a further two. For one, a cardiovascular (CVS) agent, a marginal liver weight increase was detected in primates, but was not thought to be significant as there were no histopathological or clinical chemistry changes. With another, evidence of hepatotoxicity was demonstrated in dogs at high dose levels after the clinical trials (Primates had been used rather than dogs in preclinical tests). Retrospective studies with a third compound demonstrated that the time of testing was important to identify a consistent effect on liver enzymes in dogs.

Adverse effects on the liver were not predicted for three compounds. Elevated liver enzymes were seen in less than 2% of patients with one and in more than 50% of patients with another. The third compound produced hepatic necrosis in man. Preclinical studies were examined for predictive signs, and further animal studies conducted. Neither produced additional information and it was concluded that this reaction was a human idiosyncrasy.

Discussion

For the majority of terminated compounds, development is stopped before they are evaluated in man. Cox and Styles[2] have estimated that for every 5–10,000 new compounds synthesised and screened, only 8–15 are tested in man. One of the reasons for termination at this early stage is the demonstration of overt toxicity in animal tests. There is no way of determining whether or not these compounds would have demonstrated the same toxicity in man and it is possible, therefore, that potentially useful new medicines are being lost for this reason. However, Dayan[3] stated that the rarity of predictive toxicity in man demonstrates the success of the animal toxicity procedure at preventing toxic compounds from reaching the clinic. This pilot study confirms earlier findings that only a very small proportion of compounds evaluated in volunteers and/or patients are terminated due to clinical toxicity, and nearly one-half of the side-effects causing termination are types of reaction difficult to identify in animal studies.

It is perhaps surprising that such a large proportion of these compounds were terminated due to evidence of hepatotoxicity in man, as the liver is a common target organ in animal studies. However, in animals greater emphasis is often given to histopathology findings in comparison to results obtained for clinical chemistry. In clinical testing the emphasis generally changes due to the limited opportunities for histopathology, and it is possible that greater weight is given to minor differences in clinical chemistry data. In view of the large proportion of compounds terminated due to clinical effects on the liver, a study is underway to further investigate the prediction of hepatotoxicity by animal tests.

Critique

This method of assessing the predictive value of animal studies for man has been employed in only one other published study[4] which examined important post-marketing adverse reactions to determine whether or not they had been predicted or confirmed by tests in animals.

From the data presented here, it is not possible to draw any conclusions as to why some adverse reactions were predicted and others were not. In order to do so further information would be required for each compound, such as:

- numbers of animals tested;
- animal species used;
- duration of exposure in animals and man;
- metabolism and pharmacokinetics in animals and man;
- dose levels in animals and man.

If this detailed information could be collected, this might prove to be a useful methodology for assessing the predictive value of animal studies for man.

References

1. Prentis R.A., Lis Y. and Walker S.R. (1988). Pharmaceutical innovation by the seven UK-owned pharmaceutical companies (1964-1985). *Br J Clin Pharmac.*, **25**: 387-396.
2. Cox J.S.G. and Styles A.E.J. (1979). From lead compound to product. *R & D Management*, **9**: 125-130.
3. Dayan A. (1980). The relative worth of animal testing. In: *Risk-benefit Analyses in Drug Research* (ed J.F. Cavalla) MTP Press, Lancaster, pp. 97-112.
4. Heywood R. (1984). Prediction of adverse drug reactions from animal safety studies. In: *Detection and Prevention of Adverse Drug Reactions*, Bostrom and Ljungstedt (eds). Almquist & Wiksell Int., Sweden.

7
Clinical toxicity – could it have been predicted? Post-marketing experience

RALPH HEYWOOD

Summary

1. Many adverse reactions in man, in particular immunotoxicity, allergy, hypersensitivity and effects on bone marrow, are unpredictable in animal models.
2. The correlations between target system toxicity in the rat and a non-rodent species are around 30%.
3. There is little evidence that toxicological studies have been performed with the route, dose and frequency of administration selected with due regard to the dynamics of action and target receptor sites, and with a kinetic profile that is relevant to the in-use situation. Therefore, most toxicological data cannot be interpreted.
4. The published data base is inadequate to make proper judgments, and the best guess for the correlation of adverse reactions in man and animal toxicity data is somewhere between 5% and 25%.

Introduction

Animal studies fall into two main categories: predictive evaluations of new compounds and their incorporation into schemes designed to help lessen or clarify a recognised hazard. Surprisingly, there has been little effort made to examine the qualitative predictability of human side-effects from animal studies.

Animal studies

Some analyses have attempted to assess the value of chronic animal toxicology studies[1]. The correlations between target system toxicity in the rat and a non-rodent species have been shown to be about 30%[2,3]; it is unrealistic to expect correlations between target organ toxicity in laboratory animals and adverse reactions in man to be any better. In the absence of more substantial data, one can only conclude that there is no reliable way of predicting what type of toxicity will develop in different species in response to the same compound.

Correlation of adverse reactions in man with animal toxicity data

The limited information in the literature is directed to finding correlations for specific compounds[4,5]. In a series of papers, Venning[6] identified important adverse reactions to new drugs since thalidomide. Using this list of compounds, the contributions animal studies made or could have made to the identification of these problems has been investigated[7]. An attempt has been made to update this information and the results are given here.

Table 1 lists the compounds that have been withdrawn from the British market and their main clinical adverse reactions and Table 2 classifies these compounds.

Table 1 Compounds withdrawn from the UK market for clinical adverse reactions

Year	Compounds withdrawn	Clinical adverse reactions
1980	Phenacetin	Nephrotoxicity & carcinogenicity
1981	Clioquinol	Neurotoxicity
1982	Benoxaprofen (Opren)	Skin rashes Photosensitivity Onycholysis. GI tract Fatalities in elderly
1983	Phenformin	Metabolic
	Indomethacin (Osmosin)	Small intestine perforation
	Indoprofen (Flosint)	GI tract & carcinogenicity
	Propanidid	Allergy
	Zimeldine (Zelmid)	Neurotoxicity
	Zomepirac (Zomax)	Allergy
1984	Alphaxalone	Anaphylactic shock
	Fenclofenac (Flenac)	Rashes. GI tract Carcinogenicity
	Feprazone (Methrazone)	Rashes. GI tract Thrombocytopenia Haemolytic anaemia
	Oxyphenbutazone	Haematology. GI tract
1986	Domperidone injectible (Benzamide)	Cardiotoxicity
	Guanethidine Eyedrops	Ophthalmological
	Nomifensine (Merital)	Haemolytic anaemia (Immune)
	Sulphamethoxypyridazine	Haematological Dermatological
	Suprofen (Suprol)	Reversible renal insufficiency

Table 2 Compounds withdrawn for clinical adverse reactions

Class of compound		
Anti inflammatory	Benoxaprofen (Opren)	1982
	Indomethacin-R (Osmosin)	1983
	Indoprofen (Flosint)	1983
	Feprazone (Methrazone)	1984
	Fenclofenac (Flenac)	1984
	Oxyphenbutazone	1984
	Suprofen (Suprol)	1986
Analgesics	Phenacetin	1980
	Zomepirac (Zomax)	1983
CNS		
Inhibitor of serotonin uptake	Zimeldine (Zelmid)	1983
Antidepressessant	Nomifensine (Merital)	1986
Anaesthetic	Alphaxalone	1984
	Propanidid	1983
Antidiarrhoeal	Clioquinol	1981
Antidiabetic	Phenformin	1982
Antiemetic	Domperidone injection	1986
Antihypertensive	Guanethidine (eyedrops)	1986
Antibiotic	Sulphamethoxypyridazine	1986

It can be seen that the anti-inflammatory and analgesic agents represent nearly 50% of compounds that have been withdrawn, the second most important group being the centrally active compounds, which includes anesthetics and antiemetics. Table 3 lists the major adverse reactions since 1960 and gives an assessment as to whether they were predictable from animal experimentation. Fourteen per cent of the compounds showed adverse reactions that could have been predicted.

Table 3 Major adverse reactions since 1960

		Predictable in animals
Anti-inflammatory drugs	Gastrointestinal	Yes
	Haematological	Yes
	Skin rashes	No
Alphaxalone	Anaphylaxis	No
Benoxaprofen	Fatalities, skin rashes, photosensitivity	No
Chloramphenicol	Aplastic anaemia	No
Clioquinol	Neurotoxicity	Yes
Domperidone	Cardiotoxicity	No
Halothane	Jaundice	Yes
Lincomycin, Clindamycin	Pseudomembranous colitis	No
Methysergide	Retroperitoneal fibrosis	No
Nomifensine	(Immune haemolytic anaemia)	No
Oral contraceptives	Thromboembolism	No
Phenacetin	Nephropathy	No
Phenformin	Lactic acidosis	No
Phenothiazines	Dyskinesia	Questionable
Phenylbutazone	Aplastic anaemia	No
Practolol	Oculomucocutaneous syndrome	No
Propanidid	Allergy	No
Stilboestrol	Vaginal cancer in female offspring	No (Mice)
Sulphamethoxpylidazine	Haematological dermatology	Questionable
Sympathomimetic aerosols	Asthmatic death	No
Triazolam	Amnesia	No
Zimeldine	Neurotoxicity	No

What can animal studies predict?

The current system of animal testing identifies target organ systems, several of which can be identified for a single compound. Many of the target systems identified are predictable on the basis of pharmacology. Fletcher[8] considered that 25% of toxic effects in animals might be expected as adverse reactions in man. Gastrointestinal tract intolerance carried a greater predictive capacity than many of the other effects. It would be relatively simple to extend this study and to evaluate more data retrospectively. The latest information suggests that 5% of drugs are withdrawn from clinical investigation because of predictable toxic evidence[9]. The data base we have at the moment is totally inadequate.

Lessons from specific compounds

Clioquinol

The SMON syndrome was described in Japan in the 1960s. Acute intoxication with clioquinol in dogs treated for diarrhoea was reported in 1965 and Lannek and her colleagues[10] followed up these observations. At that time, I was finding CNS damage in dogs given high doses of clioquinol in suitable dietary circumstances, though not all signs and lesions attributable to SMON were found. There is no doubt in my mind that the toxicity of clioquinol is related to absorption and that the earlier toxicological studies with the compound were carried out with the compound unabsorbed. If a compound is not bioavailable to an animal model, the study is pointless.

Contraceptive steroids

From the published toxicological data, there is no evidence either that steroids are associated with thromboembolic disease in laboratory animals, or that they induce myocardial infarction or hypertension[11]. Predictions of carcinogenicity from laboratory animals are without meaning for there is no evidence that the studies were conducted in a way that took into consideration the pharmacodynamics in the species investigated, or with any appreciation of end organ sensitivity.

NSAIDs

There is evidence of species differences, for the rat and dog are more susceptible than the monkey and guinea-pig to the gastrointestinal lesions. There is no relationship between anti-inflammatory potency and ulcerogenicity, though the degree of reduction of prostaglandin synthesis is a factor[12]. In man, dermatological and gastrointestinal signs are the most frequently recorded. Thrombocytopenia is the common blood dyscrasia; agranulocytosis or panocytopenia have been recorded and nephropathy is a common finding[13].

The kinetics of many of the NSAIDs have been investigated. Most are well absorbed and extensively bound to plasma protein. Species differences in half-life of elimination are found as are differences in the route of elimination. Often there is no metabolic transformation. These generalisations apply to the metabolism of benoxaprofen[14]. There is little evidence from any of the toxicological studies that the kinetics were taken into consideration when designing the toxicity studies. With benoxaprofen there was evidence, which was published in 1982, to show that in the elderly there were extended half-lives and slow clearance rates[15,16]. These data were available before the compound was withdrawn from market. The lesson to be learnt is that kinetics in man are more relevant than kinetics in animal models.

Analgesic nephropathy

A wide variety of analgesics and NSAIDs can cause renal papillary necrosis. Removing phenacetin from the market has not reduced significantly the incidence of this condition[17]. Analgesics such as aspirin, phenacetin, paracetamol, phenylbutazone and indomethacin do not consistently induce renal papillary necrosis in laboratory rodents; if they do so, necrosis follows high dosages. There are also problems with extra renal toxicity. Rosner[18], reviewing the problems of analgesic nephropathies in 1976, came to the conclusion that toxicologists could never have expected, foreseen or predicted, the existence of the analgesic nephropathy syndrome. All the work carried out since then would confirm this view.

Upper urethral carcinoma

A cause/effect relationship between renal papillary necrosis and upper urethral carcinomas has been suggested, but there are no confirmatory epidemiological or experimental data. In my experience of carcinogenicity studies with NSAIDs there is little evidence of carcinogenicity with any of these compounds; the only urinary tumours I am aware of are the bladder tumours recorded with paracetomol in the "Leeds" rat[19].

Practolol

Extensive toxicity studies have been performed in animals which metabolise the compound in a similar manner to man (dog, rat and mouse) and in species which metabolise the compound extensively, but no animal model has been found for the human adverse reaction[20]. It must be accepted that often there is no animal model.

Litogens or suspect litogens

Bendectin

The drug was first marketed in 1958; at the time it contained 10 mg each of doxylamine succinate (an anti-histamine with anti-nausea properties), diclomine (an antispasmodic), and pyridoxine (vitamin B6). In 1977 benedictin was reformulated to include only doxylamine and pyridoxine. There is no evidence from the review of animal data[21] that bendectin is a teratogen and, after 27 years use, the manufacturers estimated it had been used in 33 million pregnancies and there was no scientific evidence to show it to be a human teratogen. Because of controversy, adverse publicity, and law suits, the manufacturer of bendectin withdrew the product from the market. Bendectin now enters the newest category of drugs, a proven "litogen".

Danthrone

Anthraquinones are the largest group of the naturally recurring quinones. Danthrone (chrysazin) is a synthetic anthraquinone. The compound is used as a laxative. Mutagenicity of chrysazin has been reported in the Ames test (strains TA 1537 and TA 2637). Genotoxicity has been demonstrated in hepatocyte primary cultures and DNA repair tests[22]. There is evidence that chrysazin induces tumours in the intestine and liver of mice and rats[23,24]. Following warnings from the Committee on Safety of Medicines, Riker Laboratories stopped making their drug (Dorbanex), though other companies still continue to market this product, after appeal. With many million patient years experience, the decision and the basis for the decision is difficult to understand.

Conclusion

Toxicology is a science without a scientific underpinning. Animal studies are based on two assumptions; that there are appropriate animal models and that a dose-response relationship can be demonstrated. The practice of toxicology requires the administration of high (toxic) doses to animals. What hypothesis is being testing when we give to laboratory animals multiples of human doses on the basis of mg/kg body weight? There is little evidence that toxic effects observed in laboratory animals can be extrapolated through to adverse reactions to man, and "no effect" doses in animals cannot be interpreted as meaning safety. Experience would suggest, that toxicity studies are better at predicting pharmacodynamic action due to over dosage and effects due to pharmacological actions unrelated to the therapeutic use of the drug, than toxic effects. Studies conducted at maximal tolerated doses in rats and mice are labelling an increasing number of chemicals as suspect or positive rodent carcinogens. Here experience shows that apart from the anti-tumour compounds, the majority of pharmaceutical compounds (99%) that induce tumours in rodents, do so by non-genotoxic mechanisms, through physiological adaptation or as a result of direct or indirect pharmacological effects[25].

The published toxicological data are inadequate on which to base an assessment of the predictive value of animal studies for man.

References

1. Lumley C.E. and Walker S.R. (1985). The value of chronic animal toxicology studies of pharmaceutical compounds: a retrospective analysis. *Fund. Appl. Toxicol.*, **5**: 1007–1024.
2. Heywood R (1981). Target organ toxicity. *Toxicol. Lett.*, **8**: 349- 358.
3. Falahee K.J., Rose C.S., Seifried H.E. and Sawhney D. (1983). Alternatives in toxicity testing. In: *Product Safety Evaluation*, Vol 1, Ed. A.M. Goldberg. Liebert, New York. 139–162.
4. Suter K.E. (1983). Relevance of standard toxicological tests. In: *Current Problems in Drug Toxicology*. Ed. G. Zbinden, F. Cohadon, J.Y. Detaille and G. Mazue. John Libby, Paris & London. 77–89.
5. Laurence D.R., McLean A.E.M. and Wetherall M. (1984). *Safety Testing of New Drugs*. Academic Press, London.
6. Venning G.R. (1983). Identification of adverse reactions to new drugs. *Br. Med. J.*, **286**: 199–202.
7. Heywood R. (1984). Prediction of adverse drug reactions for animal studies. Skandia International Symposia. *Detection and Presentation of Adverse Drug Reactions.* pp. 173–189. Almquist and Wiksell International, Stockholm.
8. Fletcher P. (1978). Drug safety tests and subsequent clinical experience. *J. Roy. Soc. Med.*, **71**: 693–696.
9. Prentis R.A., Lis Y. and Walker S.R. (1988). Pharmaceutical innovation by 7 U.K. owned pharmaceutical companies. *Br. J. Clin. Pharmac.*, **25**: 387–396.
10. Lannek B. (1973). Toxicity of halogenated oxyquinoline in dogs: A survey of cases. *Acta Vet. Scand.*, **14**: 723–744.
11. Heywood R. (1986). An assessment of the toxicological and carcinogenic hazard of contraceptive steroids. In: *Contraceptive Steroids*. Ed. A.T. Gregoire and R.T. Blye. Plenum, New York. 231–245.
12. Rainsford K.D., Fox S.A. and Osborne D.J. (1984). Comparative effects of some NSAID on the ultrastructural integrity and prostaglandin levels in the rat gastric mucosa. *Scand. J. Gastroenterol.*, **19**: 55–68.
13. Weber J.C.P. (1984). Epidemiology of adverse reactions to NSAIDS. In: *Advances in Inflammation Research*, Vol. 6. Ed. K.D. Rainsford and G.P. Velo. Raven Press. New York. 1–7.
14. Chatfield D.H. and Green J.N. (1978). Disposition and metabolism of benoxaprofen in laboratory animals and man. *Xenobiotica*, **8**: 133–144.
15. Hamdy R.C., Murnane B, Perera N, Woodcock K. and Koch I.M. (1982). Pharmacokinetics of benoxaprofen in elderly subjects. *Eur. J. Rheumatol. Inflam.*, **5**: 69–75.
16. Kamal A. and Koch I.M. (1982). Pharmacokinetics studies of benoxaprofen in geriatric patients. *Eur. J. Rheumatol. Inflam.*, **5**: 76–81.

17. Gregg N.J., Elseviers M.M., De Broe M.E. and Bach P.H. (1989). Epidemiology and mechanistic basis of analgesic associated nephropathy. *Toxicol. Lett.*, **46**: 141-151.
18. Rosner I. (1976). Experimental analgesic nephropathy. *C.R.C. Crit. Rev. Toxicol.*, **4**: 331-352.
19. Flaks B., Flaks A. and Shaw A.P.W. (1985). Induction by paracetamol of bladder and liver tumours in the rat. *Acta Path. microbiol. Immunol. Scand.*, **93**: 367-377.
20. Reeves P.R., McCormick D.J. and Jepson H.T. (1979). Practolol metabolism in various small animal species. *Xenobiotica*, **9**: 453-458.
21. Holmes L.B. (1983). Teratogen update: Bendectin. *Teratology*, **27**: 277-281.
22. Mori H., Kawai K., Ohbayashi F., Kuniyasu T., Yamazaki M., Hamasaki T. and Williams G.M. (1984). Genotoxicity of a variety of mycotoxins in hepatocyte primary cultural/DNA repair test using rat and mouse hepatocytes. *Cancer Res.*, **52**: 2918-2923.
23. Mori H., Sugie S., Niwa K., Takahashi M. and Kawai K. (1985). Induction of intestinal tumours in rats by chrysazin. *Br. J. Cancer*, **52**: 781-783.
24. Mori H., Sugie S., Niwa K., Yoshima N., Tanaka T. and Hirono I. (1986). Carcinogenicity of Chrysazin in large intestine and liver of mice. *Jpn. J. Cancer Res.*, **77**: 871-876.
25. Heywood R. (1987). Tumour induction as a result of pharmacological effects of drugs. *NLN Publication No. 19*, 119-145.

C.
What can be Learnt from Case Studies

8
What can be learned from case studies?
The company approach

KURT E. SUTER

Summary

1. The relevance of toxicological testing can be evaluated by comparing the total numbers of correctly and falsely predicted adverse effects.
2. However, of more practical importance for the pharmaceutical industry is the correct and complete prediction of unacceptable side-effects. This can only be achieved within the safety assessment process, with a multi disciplinary approach, which has to be adapted on a case to case basis to the drug under development.
3. The retrospective evaluation of the relevance of animal studies may lead to a change in methodology, testing strategies, the decision making process and/or the organisational structure of a toxicology department.

Introduction

The relevance of toxicity studies is usually evaluated by means of retrospective comparisons (case studies) of animal and human data. Predominantly, data from repeated dose toxicity studies are used since for reproduction, mutagenicity and carcinogenicity studies the clinical data are sparse. For case studies there are two avenues that can be followed. The first is to collect data only from repeated dose studies and compare them with the corresponding clinical data (partial approach). The second is to include in the analysis supportive data which has been generated and considered within the framework of safety assessment of the drug(s) in question (holistic approach).

Both approaches have their own merits and justifications. For the efficient utilisation of the capacity of a toxicology department in terms of product safety as well as of economy, it is essential to continuously review the safety assessment process. The holistic approach is usually the method of choice.

Example of a case study

As an example of a case study a brief evaluation of six drugs developed at Sandoz is made which was presented in a more extended form at an SIR meeting[1]. Five of the drugs are still on the market: Hydergine®, Parlodel®, Sandimmun®, Zaditen® and Leponex®, whereas FK 33–824, an encephalin derivative, had to be dropped during the early clinical trial phase because of failure to pass the blood/brain barrier. The extended scope of the task made some simplifications inevitable, e.g.:

- Only distinct findings from repeated dose studies in rats and dogs were included.
- Additional experimental information was considered on a case by case basis.
- The clinical side-effects considered were those listed in the drug information provided by the manufacturer.

In respect to their relevance, animal findings can be assigned to one of four categories: correct positive findings (side-effects observed in animals as well as in patients), correct negative findings (no adverse effects in animals or patients), false positive findings (adverse effects in animals but not in patients), false negative findings (no effects in animals but in patients). Although the correct prediction of the absence of adverse effects is important, their numerical assessment is not possible, and therefore not considered in Table 1.

Table 1. Prediction of effects made for 6 Sandoz drugs in repeated dose animal studies

Category of findings	Hydergine	Parlodel	Sandimmun	Zaditen	FK 33-824	Leponex	Total findings
correct +	0	2	8	2	4	6	22
false +	6	10	7	3	12	10	48
false −	1	6	2	3	6	2	20

As can be seen from Table 1, for all 6 drugs 22 side-effects were correctly predicted in standard animal investigations (correct positive results). However, many more positive results were noted in the animal experiments than finally observed in patients. There was a total of 48 false positive results for the 6 drugs. In four cases it was possible, by means of special investigations, to demonstrate that they were irrelevant in terms of the human situation.

A total of 20 false negative results, representing 13 different types of effects, were identified in standard studies for the 6 compounds. However, in 4 cases concerning dyskinesia or aterial hypotension, the clinical effect was predicted by pharmacological investigations. The side-effects not detected in any animal experiment can be assigned to 5 groups, the greatest number concerning subjective side-effects. These are conveyed verbally, and thus are very difficult to detect in animal experiments. They are usually, however, of no particular concern. The other four categories are more serious: idiosyncratic events, and cardiovascular, CNS, and gastrointestinal effects.

General conclusions drawn from this case study

Probably the most striking finding was the great number of false predictions. This seems to confirm the doubts of all those who question animal experimentation because of a lack of predictability. However, before premature negative conclusions are drawn, some caution is advised, as indicated by the fact that 5 of the 6 drugs had already been introduced on to the market and had proved safe for patients (although in one case special risk management measures had to be taken, see below).

Serious false positive results may be interpreted as unacceptable side-effects, and consequently may lead to the unjustified rejection of promising drug candidates. In fact, for 4 of the 6 compounds there would have been good reasons for their abandonment had it not been possible to demonstrate the irrelevant nature of some of the positive findings, among them uterine neoplasms (Parlodel®), cell necrosis in peripheral tissues (Hydergine®), liver toxicity (Zaditen®), and substantial lipopigment formation in various organs (Leponex®). The great number of false positive results was mainly due to the massive overdosing that has to be practised in standard tests for hazard assessment. Furthermore, anatomical, physiological and metabolic differences between species accounted for some of these results.

For a pharmaceutical company it is of the utmost importance to have the know-how to tackle the problem of serious false positive results. Usually the problem cannot be overcome simply by a repetition of the same study, using ever more different species or strains, or by the uncritical use of ever more tests. By far the optimal way is by carrying out special investigations for the elucidation of the mechanism involved, or finding biochemical markers that can be linked to the toxic effect. Often such studies are multidisciplinary approaches involving scientists from other departments, external institutes or universities.

False negative findings represent the nightmare of any pharmaceutical company. They may ultimately lead to suffering in patients, withdrawal of the drug from the market and loss of image. It may be surprising that of the 6 compounds investigated, there were almost as many false negative findings as correct positive predictions, i.e. half of all adverse effects were correctly predicted and half were not predicted. This clearly demonstrates that the predictability of toxicological methods should not be treated as a numbers game. The primary objective of toxicological testing is to detect unacceptable side-effects rather than any adverse effect. Thus, a toxicological method that produces a relatively great number of false negative effects may still be valuable if it detects the few unacceptable side-effects. For a particular test, it is important to know what potential unacceptable side-effects cannot be detected. If the pharmacological properties or previous experience with similar drugs indicate that such effects may occur, the inclusion of additional investigations into the standard tests or the establishment of specially designed pre-screening methods, which are able to detect the effect have to be considered.

The evaluation of the relevance of toxicological tests is complicated by the fact that the decision of whether a side-effect is acceptable or not is in certain instances both extremely delicate and complex. This is demonstrated by the example Leponex®. A cluster of cases of agranulocytosis occurred in Finland. When soon afterwards rare cases of agranulocytosis were also found in other countries, the situation was considered so alarming that Sandoz Ltd. decided to remove the drug from the market. However, due to the beneficial effects of the drug, clinicians and even legislatory bodies asked the company to reconsider its decision. After a careful re-evaluation of the situation it was decided that the drug could be used under strict haematologic monitoring of the white blood cell counts. By doing so the cases of agranulocytosis diminished and marketing authorisation was granted in several countries. This example shows that under certain circumstances (when special measures are taken) even a life-threatening side-effect may not be an obstacle for the clinical use of a drug.

Practical consequences for our company

In the last few years the evaluation of case studies, particularly those of the holistic approach, has led Sandoz Ltd. to some substantial changes in the general strategy for the development of new drugs:

- The toxicological testing programme is now drafted in a joint meeting with pharmacologists, clinicians and toxicologists.
- Toxicological tailor-made prescreening methods have been developed for the early preclinical testing of certain classes of compounds.
- Various *in vitro* assays have been developed for mechanistic studies.
- Safety assessment is made in the context of exposure data such as plasma level determinations and clearance under steady state conditions, rather than dose levels applied.
- Toxicologists attend the periodical project meetings where clinical testing programmes and their results are reviewed.

The multidisciplinary safety assessment process has been further facilitated by the merger of the toxicology department, pharmacokinetics department and the human pharmacology department in a drug safety assessment department.

Outlook for the future

Millions of SFr. are being spent on ever more sophisticated tests, more sensitive analytical tools, more measurements, more specialisation, etc. However, the art of toxicology, i.e. the judgmental process has not kept pace with the rapid development of the science. There is a shortage of experts capable of linking the wealth of data from various toxicity tests and condensing and weighing the results. The transformation of specialists to become generalists is now needed. Such an attempt may be more important and less costly than constantly adding more standard tests into a given test battery.

The multi-state procedure for the marketing authorisation of new drugs as it is now in force in the EC opens up new, interesting perspectives for the assessment of the relevance of animal data. This is a formalised safety assessment procedure with defined condensation of information starting with single study reports and ending up in an expert report. Tables in a standardised form have to be prepared for each study. Filling in these tables with the support of computer programmes after completion of a study could facilitate the long-term evaluation of the relevance of toxicological test methods within a company.

Some personal thoughts

The relevance of animal experimentation can only be evaluated if adequate human data are available. Drugs which undergo extended animal testing and are given deliberately to humans represent the best opportunity for such an evaluation. Industrial toxicologists are in the privileged position of being able to take full advantage of the comprehensive information available in their companies. However, this information is either submitted under confidential cover to authorities and/or is located in archives not accessible to the scientific community.

Industrial toxicology is in great part a science of case studies. It would benefit both toxicology as well as industry if at least some of this information were made available to a greater number of scientists. As has been demonstrated particularly by case studies of the holistic approach, toxicological problems are becoming ever more complex as this field of research develops. Sometimes problems can only be solved with the help of the know how from other disciplines that are not necessarily available within a company. That it is possible to publish at least some case studies in a rather detailed manner has been demonstrated by a recent publication[2], and the CMR investigation of the value of chronic animal toxicology studies[3] is also a step in the right direction.

References

1. Suter, K.E. (1983). Relevance of standard toxicological tests: comparison of the experimental and clinical data of pharmaceutical preparations. In: *Current Problems in Drug Toxicology*, Eds. G. Zbinden, F. Dohadon, J.Y. Detaille, G. Mazue, John Libbey, Paris & London, pp.77–89.
2. Laurence, D.R., McLean, A.E.M., Weatheral, M. (1984). *Safety Testing of New Drugs*. Academic Press, 1984.
3. Lumley, C.E. and S.R. Walker (1985). The value of chronic animal toxicology studies of pharmaceutical compounds: a retrospective analysis. *Fundamental and Applied Toxicology*, **5**: 1007–1024.

9
What can be learnt from case studies? A collaborative approach

ANDRE MCLEAN

Summary

1. Several lessons can be drawn from the experience of producing a book of case studies comparing animal and clinical data:
   (i) it is possible to compile and publish detailed case studies;
   (ii) knowledge of mechanisms can be useful in demonstrating the safety of a new therapeutic candidate;
   (iii) clinical surveillance studies after marketing are important in the retrospective assessment of toxicology;
   (iv) known toxicity in man provides an opportunity to go back and determine ways of improving current methods.
2. Further studies comparing toxicology and clinical effects are needed in order to pinpoint weak aspects of toxicity testing which could lead to the destruction of potentially useful compounds.

Introduction

"Safety Testing of New Drugs"[1], which Desmond Laurence, David Weatherall and I edited a few years ago, is a compilation produced through experience and contact within the Pharmaceutical Industry, especially on the part of Desmond Laurence who was able to persuade enough companies that they would lose nothing by opening their files and making their own summary of the toxicity data and the subsequent clinical events available to a wide audience. This was done for Bethanidine (Wellcome), Bromocriptine (Sandoz), Cimetidine (SK&F), Propranolol, Practolol and Tamoxifen (ICI). The result was some comparisons of the pre-clinical and clinical toxicology for medicines which were quite successful in their times, and some which are still in widespread use.

Lessons

What lessons can can be drawn from the experience of producing this book? First of all it can be done. I do not believe any of the companies had regrets afterwards, and none of them were sued on the basis of the information that was disclosed. However it does require an enormous amount of work to dig information out of the data files, together with the trust of many companies.

The second lesson is something that has been said many times in the course of toxicology, which is that mechanisms can be very useful in demonstrating the safety of a proposed new drug in a proposed new class. This was especially true for the Sandoz contribution on Bromocriptine and the uterine tumours. If the mechanism can be identified, it can be demonstrated that a toxic effect need not be regarded as a danger signal and it can even be possible to persuade the regulatory agencies that the compound is of value and the benefit/risk ratio is in the right direction.

The third lesson is that clinical surveillance studies after marketing are of great importance in the retrospective assessment of toxicology, and this means that inside a company experience can be built up of the interaction between the toxicologist's task and subsequent events in the clinic. Of course this applies not only for the substance under study but for the whole class of drugs. Presumably it is a matter of a commercial decision on the part of individual pharmaceutical companies as to whether they are part of a scientific community and therefore share their information where possible in order to raise the general level of scientific understanding, or whether they are of the type of company where commercial secrecy takes presidence and temporary advantage over competitors is more important. From the point of view of morale and flow of information and good recruits into the company, there are advantages in openness.

The fourth lesson is that known toxicity to man provides an opportunity to look back and improve methods. Practolol is a particular example of this, although clearly no one has succeeded in finding a method which would prevent another practolol coming onto the market. Although there are many suggestions about why practolol has its effects, none have resulted in practical methods of screening out such a compound. If one worked on the basis of looking for potentially antigenic covalent protein binding, then in my opinion every new drug synthesised would be screened out.

Conclusion

The data from human and animal studies can be used together to provide an improved rationality in our risk assessment. In my opinion, more studies comparing toxicology and clinical effects are needed in order to pinpoint those aspects of our toxicology which are weak points and are liable to lead to the destruction of potentially useful compounds. We need research across drugs and we need to go back to further investigate drugs with good clinical epidemiology.

Reference

1. Laurence, D R, McLean, A E M, Wetherall M (1984). *Safety Testing of New Drugs*. Academic Press, London.

III.
Recommendations for future work: summary of discussion

10
Recommendations for future work: summary of discussion

CYNDY LUMLEY and STUART WALKER

Summary

1. Studies to assess the relevance of animal data for man are important. However, these must ensure that the animal and clinical data are comparable based on pharmacokinetic and metabolic information
2. Both retrospective studies, for which a large data base is already available, and prospective studies, where data generated using 'state of the art' methodologies are collected, should be carried out.
3. Two possible methodologies could be employed: a global approach utilising all available data, taking into account dose levels and comparing whatever is observed, and a more selective approach focused on particular types of data or phases of study.
4. Any analyses should be selective on chemical structure, pharmacological mode of action or therapeutic indication.
5. It would be of value to also establish a central register of adverse effects in animals.

Introduction

The objective of studying the correlation between animal and clinical data is to improve future predictions and risk assessment, and to pinpoint areas where basic research is needed. It is unlikely that prediction of immunologically mediated tissue changes, which are often not observed until late in clinical trials or after marketing, will be greatly improved by this type of study. However, useful information can be obtained in relation to adverse effects related to known pharmacological activity, secondary pharmacological effects, and direct tissue damage which should all be detectable in animals.

It must be accepted that the relevance of major animal toxicity for man is unprovable, apart from special cases such as medicines for life-threatening conditions and antineoplastic agents. Where animal toxicity has occurred, but study in man was still permitted, the predictive value is good and this may be an area where greater emphasis should be placed on human studies. The occurrence of serious adverse effects in man, which were unanticipated from the animal data, implies poor predictive value and future studies should address ways in which this can be improved.

Comparability of animal and clinical data

Any study designed to assess the relevance of animal tests for man must ensure that the animal and clinical data are comparable based on pharmacokinetic and metabolic information. There is a relatively limited number of medicines for which good human pharmacokinetic and metabolic data and similar animal data are available, and where there has been exposure of humans and animals under comparable conditions. There is a difficulty, however, in establishing the correct parameters upon which to base an assessment of comparability: parent compound or metabolite(s), steady state or peak blood levels, target organ exposure, differences in sensitivity. Setting these criteria too strictly will limit the amount of data available for comparison. In any case, evidence of absorption in both species is essential, and pharmacokinetic and metabolic data are important in the interpretation of the results of these comparisons.

Retrospective or prospective studies

Both retrospective and prospective studies are needed. The advantage of retrospective studies is that a large amount of information is already available, and these can therefore, be carried out over a fairly short time period. Any information collected in this way should be limited to the post-GLP period, and pharmacokinetic and metabolic data must be included. One possible approach would be to use the results of a retrospective study to construct guidelines that could be validated using a prospective approach.

Prospective studies have the advantage of collecting data generated using 'state of the art' methodologies, and can be carried out with a specific objective. This type of study would enable an assessment of predictions made at each stage of the drug development process without the bias of hindsight. For example, it should be possible to collect information on compounds for which toxicity in animals caused some concern at the time when the decision was taken to go into man, and then collect the clinical data as it becomes available.

Global or selective approach

A global approach, where all available data is utilised and comparisons of all observations are made, has been employed for retrospective studies. However, the large amount of information collected can result in difficulties with interpretation and inevitably generalisations and assumptions must be made. These problems could be avoided by using a more selective approach, focussing on particular types of data or phases of study. Suggestions for selective studies include:

1. separating acute and chronic effects;

2. limiting clinical data to that obtained in healthy human volunteers;
3. collecting biochemical and functional test data only;
4. focussing on toxicity in animals that did not prevent compounds from being taken into man;
5. focussing on serious clinical toxicity.

Central register of animal effects

A central register of drug-related toxicity in animals might enable the identification of trends within specific chemical, therapeutic or pharmacological classes, which could be beneficial to the pharmaceutical industry in interpretation of animal data. Animal adverse reactions could be reported anonymously in a similar way to the yellow card system. Relevant information about each compound, animal husbandry and environmental conditions would also have to be collected for this database to be of value.

Conclusion

Several questions must be addressed in any study proposal for comparing animal and clinical data, including:

1. How can data transfer between clinical and basic science be improved?
2. Who has the responsibility of carrying out the additional animal follow-up studies?
3. Who will ultimately utilise the data, and will the regulators pay any attention to it?

Comparative studies of animal and clinical data could be valuable in improving prediction of adverse effects related to known pharmacological action, secondary pharmacological action or direct toxic effects, particularly in reducing the incidence of serious effects in man which were unanticipated from the animal data. Both retrospective and prospective

Recommendations for Future Work: Summary of Discussion

studies should be undertaken in parallel, utilising a selective approach focussed on particular types of data or phases of study. Evidence of absorption in both animals and man is essential, and pharmacokinetic and metabolic data are important in the interpretation of the results.

Index

Anthracycline 30
Antineoplastic 23, 30
Asparaginase 30
Aspirin 63

Benoxaprofen 53, 59, 60, 61, 63
Bethanidine 80
Bleomycin 29
Bromocriptine (Parlodel) 72, 73, 74, 80

Carcinogenicity 3, 7, 8, 9, 10, 11, 29, 38, 59, 61, 62, 63
  prediction of 8, 12, 43, 54, 59
  tests 7, 8, 9, 10, 12, 31, 36, 38, 55, 64
Case studies 63, 64, 65, 69, 71, 72, 73, 74, 79
Cimetidine 80
Clinical toxicity 47, 49, 51, 53, 54, 57
Clioquinol 53, 54, 59, 60, 61, 62
Committee on Safety of Medicines (CSM) 41, 42, 44, 65

Data base 7, 11, 15, 16, 26, 36, 57, 62
Dorbanex 65

Fertility 24
  testing 42

Gastrointestinal
  epithelium 24

intolerance 28, 61
lesions 62
toxicity 26, 28, 59, 74
Genotoxicity 8, 64
  tests 12

Hydergine 72, 73, 74

Immunotoxicity 6, 57
Indomethacin 59, 63

Kidney(s) 11
  renal toxicity 23, 27, 29, 59, 63

Leponex 72, 73, 74, 75
Liver
  enzymes 11, 53, 54
  hyperplasia 11
  necrosis 4, 54
  toxicity 23, 27, 29, 49, 54, 55, 74
  tumours 10, 11, 65

Mechanism(s) 16, 18, 65, 74, 79
Mutagenicity 7, 44, 64
  studies 8, 11, 72

Nalidixic acid 43

Paracetamol 63, 64
Pharmacokinetic(s) 45, 55, 76
  data 6
  studies 3, 4
Pharmacology 61, 76
  studies 4, 6
Phenacetin 60, 62, 63

Phenformin 43, 60, 61
Phenylbutazone 61, 63
Practolol 43, 45, 61, 80
Prediction 7, 8, 16, 18, 23, 24, 25, 26, 27, 29, 49, 51, 54, 55, 57, 62, 71
  false negative 26, 27, 31, 73, 75
  false positive 9, 23, 27, 73, 74
  true positive 26, 27, 73
Predictive value 14, 18, 23, 24, 27, 50, 58, 65
Propranolol 80

Reactions
  idiosyncratic 54, 74
  immune 4, 5, 35, 57, 60, 62
  life threatening 26, 76
Risk assessment 4

Salbutamol 43
Sandimmun 72
Spironolactone 43
Streptozotocin 29

Studies
  investigative 18
  prospective 15, 16, 23, 24, 25, 35
  retrospective 15, 16, 23, 24, 25, 26, 33, 34, 35, 37, 38, 42, 43, 46, 54, 62, 71, 72, 79

Tamoxifen 80
Thalidomide 43, 58
Thiourea 11
Toxicokinetics 45

Zaditen 72, 73, 74